MISCARRIED

joy

TANIKA FITZGERALD

MISCARRIED JOY
Moving Beyond Incredible Pain to Extraordinary Faith

Published by:
NyreePress Literary Group
Fort Worth, TX 76161
1-800-972-3864
www.nyreepress.com

Cover designed by Willie Blue

Scripture verses marked NLT are taken from the NEW LIVING TRANSLATION. Scripture verses marked AMP are taken from the AMPLIFIED BIBLE. Scripture verses marked KJV are taken from the KING JAMES VERSION of the BIBLE. Scripture verses marked MSG are taken from THE MESSAGE TRANSLATION. Scripture verses marked CEV are taken from the CONTEMPORARY ENGLISH TRANSLATION. Scripture verses marked NKJV are taken from the NEW KING JAMES VERSION of the BIBLE.

ISBN 13: 978-1-945304-15-6

Library of Congress Control Number: 2016958869

Religion/Christian Life/Women's Issues

Printed in the United States of America

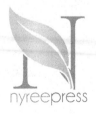

nyreepress

Acknowledgements

To God: I wondered why miscarriage was part of my journey to motherhood (which I know will manifest soon). I definitely would not have chosen this journey and there were times when I wanted to give up. But then you whispered to me, "Use your pain for My purpose," so here we are. Thank You for covering this project with your love and for opening up opportunities for my story to touch the lives of women all over the world.

To my husband: you have been a solid rock in every loss. Thank you for caring for me, praying for me and standing in faith with me. The tears you wiped from my eyes were countless and I know that I was able to endure because you held me in your arms and in your heart. You are going to make an awesome father and I can't wait to witness you sharing your love with our children. Your sacrifice while I was writing this book did not go unnoticed. This is our book, baby!

To my parents: There simply isn't another father and mother like you on this earth. Your love, support and dedication to your children is incomparable. You have been there throughout our losses. Thank you for carrying me when I didn't know how to stand, for wiping my tears, for traveling just for hugs and quality time together. I couldn't have overcome these obstacles without you and I will be forever grateful for all you have done. I haven't encountered any challenges where you weren't there for me. You have been there for every celebration in my life and I can't wait to celebrate the day when you will officially become Papa and Gran Gran!

To my Sisters: You were my first children (in my mind). You have no idea how often I prayed for you before God even formed you in mom's womb. I was ecstatic the day that you were born and it has been a journey of joy from that day forward. Your very existence increases my faith because I know all that mom went through physically and emotionally for you to be here. It increases my faith to a level that is unexplainable. What God did for mom and dad, He will do for me. Thank you for your love, support, prayers and faith as you await to become aunties ready to spoil your nephews and nieces.

To My Sands: To know that you will drive or fly any distance to be there for love, support, hugs and tears further lets me know that you are God's blessing and His extended arms for me here on earth. I appreciate your prayers, your encouragement and your love. We were Especially Made to Endure Never Ending Trials and we do it well!

To Buddy: Everyone needs a girlfriend that will laugh or cry with them on the spot! That is certainly you. It's unexplainable but we truly feel what each other is going through. You have no idea how your morning calls encouraged me to stay faithful in knowing that God will bring forth our children in His timing. Your encouragement in this waiting season is the best gift! Life is a colorful array of beautiful flowers because I have you in mine.

To Tiffany: You are the friend and sister who always brings sunshine to a rainy day and the life to any party. Thank you for the prayers you take to the feet of Jesus on my behalf in your quiet time with Him. Your love, support and friendship mean the world to me and I am blessed to have you in my life. I pray for you just like you pray for me.

To Sheila: I did not know the power of an accountability partner in this journey until I had you as mine. Thank you for your help in keeping me focused, checking on me daily and even offering to whisk me away when I needed it. I pray that what you poured into me during my long process of writing this book is returned to you more than one-hundred fold. I pray you are blessed with an immense amount of success in all you do. Your accountability has been a blessing that simply cannot be put into words.

To Kennisha Thornton & the Nyree Press Staff: Thank you for helping my dream come true. Working with you has been such a joy, not to mention seamless. I am beyond pleased with my decision to self-publish with Nyree Press.

To LaKeisha Rainey-Collins: Thank you for your great attention to detail through the editing process of my book. You helped to make *Miscarried Joy* even better for my readers. Your heart is amazing and your gift is appreciated.

Dedication

This book is dedicated to my 3 angel babies. Although I never met you nor gave you all names, I carry you in my heart and my life is forever changed because you once existed. I will meet you in heaven!

Foreword

When my daughter asked me to write the foreword for her book I was honored, yet sad. The very painful memories resurfaced, those memories of the miscarriages she experienced and the grandbabies I lost. As a mother, you bear the pains and sufferings of your children. I relived these moments, in my head and in my heart. Even though there's sadness, there is joy. Watching the strength of my daughter and the faith she has in God even through all that she has been through has helped me to accept these situations with thanksgiving.

Although many of her friends are having children and the baby shower invites are rolling in one after the other, her faith has not wavered. I admire how she has been able to smile, love and support her friends, attend the showers, and very truly be happy and excited for them. The way I see her celebrate others is beyond remarkable. Tanika and her husband have even agreed to be Godparents to some.

Tanika displays God's love in so many ways. Her faith in Him is evident and her ability to still believe even through adversity displays an uncommon level of strength. She is so giving and it's for this reason she is sharing her experiences to help others that may not know how to handle the hurt and pain that comes along with losing a child.

"For I consider that the sufferings of this present time are not worthy to be compared with the glory which shall be revealed in us." (Romans 8:18 NKJV)

In my heart I see nothing but favor, blessings and God's glory in my daughter's life. I confidently declare that she will be granted every desire that lies in the depth of her heart. I pray daily that God will reward her for her selflessness, for her faithfulness and most of all for never losing sight of His role in her life. We give glory to God as we wait in faith for the conception and birth of my grandchildren. I cannot wait to meet them, love them and spoil them, of course! Tanika will be an awesome mother!

I pray that after reading this book, your faith in God will be increased and you will love Tanika just as much as I love her.

Deborah Jones
(Tanika's Mother)

Table of Contents

**Part One:
Understanding God's Heart
in the Midst of Incredible Pain**

**Part Two:
Faith-Building Lessons from Barren Women**

Part Three:
Walking in Extraordinary Faith

Part One

Understanding God's Heart in the Midst of Incredible Pain

Prelude

My Miscarried Joy

First comes love, then comes marriage and then comes the baby in the baby carriage. Isn't that what we sang as little girls? Isn't that the dream that was placed in our hearts for as long as we could remember? Well, it was for me. As a little girl, I dreamed about the day I would meet my prince charming. I longed for the day my father would escort me down the aisle wearing a gorgeous white gown, tears filling my eyes as I gazed at my very soon-to-be husband. We would live happily ever after and definitely be fruitful and multiply. It would happen *just like that!* What never entered my mind was the possibility of it being difficult to successfully conceive and carry a baby full term. I had heard of many women experiencing miscarriages, still birth, barrenness or other complications, but it never once entered my mind that *I* would share in any of these. Nope, not Tanika. I was going to conceive easily, have easy pregnancies, carry my healthy babies to term and bounce back with no issues at all. That was *my* plan. Now, let me share with you what real life was like for my husband Maurice, and I.

We stopped our method of birth control six months after our wedding. We were ready to enter into one of the hardest, yet most rewarding roles on earth - parenthood. We actually didn't think about when we would get pregnant, nor did we implement any methods to speed up conception. We just had lots of fun, if you know what I mean! Shortly after returning from vacation in Florida, Maurice told me that he thought I was pregnant. I laughed hysterically because I was certain he was wrong. So, my husband being the curious man he is, went to get a pregnancy test to prove me wrong. Me, having the certainty I had, took the test to show him that he was wrong. Boy, did I have to swallow my words that day!

On June 8, 2015, we were filled with incredible joy as a positive result was revealed on our pregnancy test. We laughed, we cried and our hearts were instantly filled with an unexplainable love for the child who was growing in my belly. Besides the day I accepted Christ and married my husband, this was one of the best feelings of my life. I was becoming a mother! Maurice and I instantly went to a level of prayer that we had not before. Daily, he prayed over my womb and I changed my eating habits and physical activity. It was no longer about me. The baby I was carrying became a top priority. We are very close to our family, so waiting twelve weeks to let the cat out of the bag was not an option. We delivered the exciting news to our parents and siblings. From that day, our lives were changed. The decisions I made from that day affected another life instantly. I made any required changes to ensure that the life and health of my child was in the best state possible.

Then, the unthinkable happened. On June 21, 2015, which happened to be Father's Day, at seven weeks pregnant, I got the scare of my life. I began to bleed and it would not stop. I called the doctor and heard the words no woman with child wants to hear: *"You are probably beginning to miscarry and there is nothing that I can do about it."* I could not hold back the tears. I informed my husband and he instantly began to pray. I was so thankful for his level of faith that day, because all I could hear was "miscarriage" but he refused to accept it. So we joined in faith – believing everything was going to be fine. Days went by and the bleeding had not stopped. Blood tests confirmed my greatest fear – we had lost our baby.

My world, which had quickly been filled with joy just a few weeks prior, was instantly filled with a level of incredible pain. Why was this happening to me? What did I do to cause this? What did I do to deserve this pain? Why would God allow me to get pregnant and then allow me to miscarry? These are just some of the questions I asked myself. I wasn't ready to talk to the doctor about next steps. I wanted to hear from God about why this was happening to us. I wanted Him to tell me why and how such happiness could be taken away from us so abruptly. Maurice was my pillar of strength when I had none. We had to break the news to our parents and siblings and then make a decision on what process we would use to clear the womb. To me, I was carrying life but to the doctors, I was carrying just a fetus. I was emotionally connected to my baby and the thought of having to undergo a forty-five-minute procedure to "extract" a baby that we were lovingly connected to was overwhelming.

On July 6th, the day of my dilation and curettage, I cried thinking about what had occurred in my body. My husband

I am to *rejoice* in

my tribulations – not

because I like *pain* –

but because God is

using life's *difficulties*

and Satan's attacks to

build my *character*.

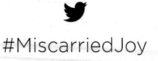

#MiscarriedJoy

and I had conceived a life and that life had come to an end inside of me. I dreaded each step I took as I walked towards the operating room. The thought of waking up with an empty womb that once held my very first child is unexplainable. My husband was amazing through this whole process and had it not been for him, I would not have made it through with my faith in tact and still trusting God.

A few days following the procedure, I received a call from my doctor. I could instantly hear a high level of concern in her voice. A greater level of fear hit my spirit as I heard her say "You need to get here immediately. Your blood work shows that you are *still* pregnant. We need to find out where that other baby is and I don't want to take a chance of your tubes bursting." I instantly hung up the phone, packed up my things, called my husband and headed to the hospital. My nerves were a wreck as I went from one ultrasound to the next, from the doctor's office to the hospital, to more blood work, to multiple pelvic exams. During the final ultrasound, the technician located another baby on my ovary. Yes, I was carrying twins! I had experienced a heterotopic pregnancy - the existence of two (or more) simultaneous pregnancies with separate implantation sites, one of which is ectopic.

In the midst of my healing, I again felt that unbearable pain, but this time, it was from the reality of losing two babies. Following this discovery, I received medication through multiple injections to dissolve the remaining fetus from my body. I had to have blood work taken every week for 6 weeks following the injections. It was one of the most emotional times of my life. I was reminded of my loss every week for a total of eight weeks. The healing process was difficult to say the least.

All of my family and friends perceive me as a pillar of strength and because of that, I felt that I needed to convey I was okay. But secretly, I was in a whirlwind of an emotional battle. I became depressed and I was disappointed with God. I was crushed. Broken. Empty. Hurt. I felt like my female body should be able to do what God designed it to do with no issues. I blamed myself and I blamed God. As I spent time in prayer and studying God's Word, I was reminded of the following scripture:

> *"Dear brothers and sisters, when* **troubles of any kind** *come your way,* **consider it an opportunity for great joy.** *For you know that when your* **faith is tested,** *your* **endurance has a chance to grow.** *So let it grow, for when your endurance is fully developed, you will be perfect and complete, needing nothing." (James 1:2-4)*

This scripture was packed with everything I needed to walk in my healing. I was finally able to accept that there was nothing I did to cause the miscarriage. I was experiencing trouble with a purpose. I am to rejoice in my tribulations – not because I like pain – but because God is using life's difficulties and Satan's attacks to build my character. God had allowed this suffering to hit our lives to deepen our trust in Him. Rather than drowning in my disappointments, I chose to immerse in God's Word. I chose to trust His timing regarding children and every other desire for our lives. We walked in our healing and continued to live and enjoy life, while healing from the pain. We stood in faith and remained mindful that we can make many plans, but the Lord's purpose will prevail (Proverbs 19:21). Having children is one of our deepest desires and we

Getting beyond

incredible pain

will not be easy,

but my *faith* will

make it *possible*.

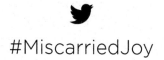

#MiscarriedJoy

firmly believe that God will bring forth our children in His timing. Therefore, we chose not to plan children, but rather to just let another pregnancy happen in His perfect timing. And it did.

On October, 29, 2015, just 4 days after our one-year anniversary, an incredible joy filled our hearts once again. It was a pleasant surprise to see a positive result on the pregnancy test. The hours slowly passed by as I impatiently waited for Maurice to get home so I could tell him the good news in a very creative and fun way. His eyes filled with tears as he opened a box to find baby shoes inside of his along with a positive pregnancy test. We were definitely ready for this journey and with our faith, we were assured that this baby would come forth with no complications.

The very next day I wrote our confession for a healthy pregnancy, a healthy baby and a supernatural, pain free birth. That was the level of our faith. I called the doctor and our first appointment was set. A few weeks later, filled with excitement, we made our way to the doctor's office for our first ultrasound. We could not wait to see our third child on the screen. The doctor confirmed that the pregnancy had made it to my uterus. Everything was just fine and thus, it was time to celebrate! We decided to keep the news a secret until Thanksgiving when all of our family would be together. That would be the perfect day to share the news.

Our second appointment was scheduled the week prior to Thanksgiving. This was the day we would get to hear our baby's heartbeat. But it didn't quite happen that way. As I laid on the table glaring at the ultrasound screen, I could see a look of concern on the technician's face.

"Is everything okay?" I asked. She responded "I can't find the fetus and your gestational sac is irregular." My heart immediately sank into my stomach and tears filled my eyes. "Not again, God," I cried. Maurice's faith went into action as he said, "Well, we can come back next week and everything will be just fine." I honestly wasn't as convinced. So another week went by and we returned to the doctor's office for another ultrasound. To my surprise, there was my baby!

We could see the fetus just as clear, although the technician still looked concerned and confused at the same time. "The fetus is there, but it is very small and your sac is still irregular." As she left the room to get the doctor, Maurice and I immediately began to pray. What was an empty sac a week prior now held our precious bundle of joy. Though the measurements were behind the doctor's original calculation and the sac was irregular, something had happened through our prayers over the past week.

The doctor returned and she, too, was confused. She requested we wait another week to see what would happen. Her words prior to leaving the room were "I do want to prepare you with news that this pregnancy may not be viable." We heard her, but it was time to put our faith in action and remove any doubt regarding our confession of a healthy pregnancy. A week and a half passed by before our next appointment. Another Wednesday meant another ultrasound for us. Again, I glared at the ultrasound screen and everything looked the same. I immediately knew that I had gained another angel baby before we heard the sad words, "I can't find the heartbeat." So at nine weeks pregnant, we lost another baby.

In the midst of this news, I was planning a baby shower for my cousin. It was incredibly difficult to celebrate a baby when I had *just* lost mine. I knew God was using this celebration to remind me that He is no respecter of persons and one day, many of our loved ones would come together to celebrate the coming birth of our child. In the midst of our mourning, I had to obey God and *"rejoice with those that rejoice" (Romans 12:15).*

On December 11, 2015, I was at the same hospital with the same staff going through the same procedure to extract the body of the fetus whose soul had already went to be with The Lord. Another dreadful walk into the same operating room with a deeper level of pain than the first time, waking up to an empty womb once again while gaining another angel baby. Although our three babies never entered this world, their footprints will forever be engraved in our hearts.

My spirit was crushed and I am unable to explain what happened to my faith in that moment. I was angry, hurt and honestly, the last thing I wanted to do was pray or read the Bible. I didn't want to hear my husband talk about his faith, God's timing or say those words that I despised in this moment, "Everything happens for a reason." Really? Well what was the reason for losing a third child? Where was God in that? We had been through so much in 2015. To end the year with this loss was devastating for me. I felt like Job! I felt as if the very thing that I wanted was snatched from me again. I was secretly ready to give up on having children. I allowed the enemy to temporarily choke my faith in God and to

Through my *prayers*,

I invited Christ to make

His *home* in the depths

of my hurting *heart*; to

strengthen my faith, my

trust, my *confidence*,

and my hope.

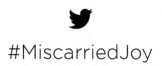

#MiscarriedJoy

doubt His promises. I questioned if I would ever be able to bear children.

Thoughts of never being able to give my husband a son entered my mind. I told everyone I was okay, but the truth was that I was suffering in silence. I cried every day for weeks. I didn't want to be angry with God, but I was. I didn't have any words for prayer so I would just sit in His presence and cry. I didn't unveil my emotions with anyone until that day when my mother called. Mothers always seem to know just what to say. My mother could hear the pain in my voice. I finally broke down. I remember her saying this to me:

"Tanika, you and Maurice will have healthy children! You know God and you know His Word. Don't you allow this disappointment to crumble your faith in Christ. This too shall pass and one day soon, you will be holding your precious babies in your arms."

In that moment, I was fully reminded of God's promises concerning children. I accepted that this was just another milestone on my journey to becoming a mother. God was creating the perfect setting for a miracle to take place in our lives. This was the beginning of my healing journey and as I write this book, God is still mending the broken pieces of my heart. I knew the only way to heal, with my faith in God being greater than it has ever been, was to seek the comfort only He could provide. In my quiet time with God, I repeatedly asked Him, "Why me?" I was honest with my feelings. I poured out everything that was in my thoughts and on my heart. Lord, why was this life given to me? He answered, "Because you are strong enough to live it."

The strength that God gives comes through the journey of our trials, and this was mine. It was not easy to get through and we are still healing. But we still believe and stand strong in faith that we will have healthy children in God's perfect timing. We have experienced incredible pain and are now on the journey towards extraordinary faith.

The journey has not been easy and honestly, this isn't one I thought I would ever have to travel. But God, in His sovereignty and perfection, has a plan that is beyond anything I can imagine. There were moments where I just could not see myself on the other side of this mountain - healed, restored and still trusting God. I had to come to the realization that my miscarriages were not God's fault. This was an attack of the enemy to destroy our trust, faith and hope in Christ.

In the months following the second miscarriage, I felt so broken; I felt as if the pieces of my heart had been scrambled on the floor and I did not know where to start in piecing them together again. I could barely see through the tears to begin the process of restoration. Then I realized that each tear of sadness, frustration and disappointment was essential to my healing. My healing began in my obedience to write this book for women like you and me.

MY HEALING

In my brokenness, I ran to God! I knew that to prevent from moving into a state of sadness and depression, I needed a level of comfort I could only find in His presence. I searched the scriptures to keep my faith intact. I read about every barren woman in The Word and my faith was ignited when I noticed something I already knew – something that was especially profound in this particular season of my life – most of these women went on to have the children they desired! That was the moment I stopped dwelling on what happened, made the decision to heal from this pain and began my journey towards extraordinary faith for God to manifest our children here on earth!

The testing of faith produces perseverance (James 1:3). I stood firmly on the promise that the God of hope would fill me with joy and peace as I trust in Him, so that I would overflow with hope by the power of the Holy Spirit (Romans 15:13). I knew I could not allow my faith to dwindle because it would be impossible to please Christ without solid faith in Him (Hebrews 11:1). As a child of the Most High King, I had to look beyond my current circumstances and focus on what He is able to do, because I live by faith and not by sight (2 Corinthians 5:7). Getting beyond the incredible pain we experienced would not be easy, but my faith would make it possible.

I can't think of one person who would raise their hands to God and say, "Lord, choose me to experience trials, challenges, loss, despair or the like." I have news for you. That is exactly what we do when we accept Christ as our Lord and Savior.

"And since we are His children, we are His heirs. In fact, together with Christ we are heirs of God's glory. But if we are to share His glory, we must also share His suffering." (Romans 8:17)

There is a price for being a follower of Jesus - you have to endure suffering, pressures of various kinds, persecution and some even face death for following Christ. James informs us of this:

"When troubles of any kind come your way, consider it an opportunity for great joy. For you know that when your faith is tested, your endurance has a chance to grow. So let it grow, for when your endurance is fully developed, you will be perfect and complete, needing nothing." (James 1:2-4)

My miscarried joy, who are now my angels in heaven, were part of my journey of suffering for Christ and are my stepping-stones to walking in extraordinary faith. The enemy asked God if he could test me and God allowed it, but He did not cause it. To share in the glory of Christ, I must also share in His suffering. *But because I have been justified through faith, I have peace through Jesus Christ (Romans 5:1).* Nothing I suffer will ever compare to the great price Jesus paid for our sins and salvation through His crucifixion and resurrection. Jesus came to the earth to die for all people. When He was crucified, so were our worries, our fears, our doubts and our anxiety. Paul informs us that suffering will be a part of life and we cannot choose the tests that will lead to our testimonies.

*Because of Christ and our faith in him, we can now come boldly and confidently into God's presence. So please **don't*** *lose heart because of my trials here. I am suffering for you, so you should feel honored. When I think of all this, I fall to my knees and pray to the Father, the Creator of everything in heaven and on earth. I pray that from his glorious, unlimited resources he will empower you with inner strength through his Spirit. Then Christ will make his home in your hearts as you trust in him. Your roots will grow down into God's love and keep you strong. And may you have the power to understand, as all God's people should, how wide, how long, how high, and how deep his love is. May you experience the love of Christ, though it is too great to understand fully. Then you will be made complete with all the fullness of life and power that comes from God. Now all glory to God, who is able, through his mighty power at work within us, to accomplish infinitely more than we might ask or think. (Ephesians 3:12-20)*

I could not allow my present troubles to get me down. I had to get down on my knees, as often as I needed, to ask for strength to endure and to overcome. Through my prayers, I invited Christ to make His home in the depths of my hurting heart; to strengthen my faith, my trust, my confidence and my hope. My doubts and fears were eliminated. In my healing process, I experienced a deeper love of Christ. I thought about Him hanging on the cross just for me. If He would do that, then surely, He can do this! His arms outstretched was an expression of His love for me. He hung high and the cross went deep into the ground - all for me. When I think about all Jesus did on the earth before His death, I am thoroughly convinced that my suffering pales in comparison to His sacrifice on the cross. As much as the losses hurt, I know victory belongs to me because of His great sacrifice and love.

I now know part of the purpose of losing our babies was because God wanted to use me to equip and encourage women who have experienced pregnancy loss to stand in faith, believing that God will do what you desire, according to your faith. Every calling comes with a cost and this was part of mine. My husband and I continue to confess what we believe for - healthy, full-term pregnancies resulting in healthy children. We cannot allow the enemy to influence us to give up on our dreams of having children.

> *"The thief comes only in order to steal and kill and destroy. I came that they may have and enjoy life, and have it in abundance [to the full, till it overflows]." (John 10:10 AMP)*

Satan's role in the earth is to test our faith, ultimately get us out of the will of God and off the path which leads to His perfect plan. The enemy was only doing what he came to do - to steal, kill and destroy. When I read this scripture over and over again, it prompted me to ask God about my role in this situation. His response is found in Mark 11:24. *"For this reason I am telling you, whatever things you ask for in prayer [in accordance with God's will], believe [with confident trust] that you have received them, and they will be given to you" (AMP)*. We still believe God and we patiently await the manifestation of His promise for us to be fruitful and multiply.

> *"Then God blessed them and said, "Be fruitful and multiply. Fill the earth and govern it. Reign over the fish in the sea, the birds in the sky, and all the animals that scurry along the ground." (Genesis 1:28)*

As I write this book, tears are filling my eyes. I still feel a mixture of emotions when I think about my journey to motherhood being more challenging than I ever imagined. I am sure some of you reading this may have experienced multiple miscarriages, stillbirth or even infertility. I penned this book just for you. I want you to know that in the midst of your doubts, fears, cries, frustrations and temptation to give up, God is still God. He is able to do the impossible. Don't stop believing and don't stop confessing. We shall have what we say, and one day we will look our beautiful babies in the eyes with an undying love and appreciation for them. You and I have the perfect setting for a miracle to take place in our lives. It will come to pass when we get beyond the incredible pain and walk in our extraordinary faith. Let's journey down this road together.

Introduction

*"Let your hope make you glad. Be patient in
time of trouble and never stop praying."
(Romans 12:12 CEV)*

Many women dream of becoming wives and then mothers. The thought of holding a precious bundle of joy you carried for nine months is an unexplainable feeling. You don't think of the possible challenges; you simply think of the outcome – holding your perfect and beautiful baby whom God knew before He formed them in the womb. You anxiously look forward to this experience and all that comes along with it. I bet those barren women in the bible had this same excitement after they got married. I bet they looked forward to giving their husbands sons and daughters to complete their family. But what about those women who struggled with making their dreams come true?

Sarah, Rebekah, Rachel, Elizabeth and Hannah - these are women I connect with in a deep way. I'd like to call them my friends, better yet, my mentors in this specific area of my life. They each share the very same trial and successfully

Some of our *tests*

come to strengthen our faith,

some come to *strengthen*

our relationship with God and

some come so we can help others

to *overcome* the same things

we have experienced.

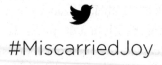

#MiscarriedJoy

overcame the trick from the enemy - barrenness. Each of these women had the very heartbeat of a mother before their deep desire was physically manifested in the earth. Sarah was said to be too old to bear a child. Rebekah, after many attempts to conceive, remained barren. Rachel so desperately yearned for a child that she gave her maid, Bilhah, to Jacob to give him the son that she could not. Elizabeth and her husband Zechariah were well beyond the child bearing years and still barren. Hannah is probably the most known woman in the bible who desperately yearned for a son of her very own. There were numerous women in biblical times who battled infertility. During these days, the highest value of a woman was placed first on her virginity and after marriage, her ability to reproduce.

A woman who could not give her husband a child was deemed as useless. There weren't any fertility clinics they could visit to provide assistance for their condition and the technology that exists today certainly wasn't available in those days. All they could do was pray and wait, or take matters into their own hands by having their maidservant bear children with their husbands, which a few did. I find it very interesting that almost every barren woman mentioned in the bible eventually conceived and birthed a healthy child. So I asked myself, If God has done it for so many women in these days, *why wouldn't He do it for me? God is no respecter of persons and He does not show favoritism (Romans 2:11).*

You probably picked up this book because you are a modern day Sarah, Rachel, Elizabeth, Rebekah or Hannah. You may be currently battling with infertility or have experienced the loss of a child through miscarriage, stillbirth or premature death.

As you read the words on these pages, we are connecting as a family of women who yearn so deeply for something God has not yet manifested in our lives. I know the pain you feel, the disappointment you've endured, the hurt and the emotional roller coaster you've had to ride in this journey. It simply cannot be put into words. You may be a woman who has an intimate relationship with God and now you feel like He has stripped away your greatest joy. Maybe you are a woman who is still growing in your relationship with God and now, because of your loss, you question how much God truly loves you. Maybe you doubt He will bring forth your desire for children in the earth. Maybe you don't have a relationship with Christ and due to your loss, you are no longer interested in developing your spiritual trust in a God you think would cause so much pain in your life. Whichever category you fit into, I wrote this book for you, I experienced my loss for you and God is using my pain to serve you.

Often times, our eyes become clouded in the midst of pain and disappointment in our lives. We focus on the hurt and question why we were chosen to endure these trials and tribulations. This is surely how I feel whenever I experience pain in my life. I am the type of person who wants to know the reason for everything and I aim to understand what God wants me to learn in and from the situation. I have repeatedly asked God, "Lord, why me?"

Some of our tests come to strengthen our faith, some come to strengthen our relationship with God and some come so we can help others to overcome the same things we have experienced. After losing our third child, I asked God, "Lord, why was this journey given to me?" He again whispered, "Because you are strong enough to handle it." As I

The only thing worse

than losing the

greatest joy

of your life is

pretending as

if you lost nothing.

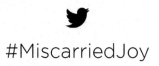

#MiscarriedJoy

prayed through my pain, God nudged me to write this book to help women who are suffering in silence. Women like you. Many women experience miscarriage or infertility without their family or close friends having one inkling of the loss that occurred or their inability to conceive. They cover it up and never speak of it as if it is taboo. It is the very reason why most women wait twelve weeks to share the news of a coming bundle of joy. What is really happening is we are operating in a spirit of fear - fear that the joy you are carrying won't physically manifest in the earth. If something does happen, you won't ever have to reveal to anyone that you *were* expecting.

Miscarriage is death. I know that's hard to hear, but it's an unfortunate reality. You miscarry a bundle of joy, but there aren't any bereavement days, no sick days and you may feel pressured to move on as if nothing has happened. You hear about how common it is and some will even say, depending on how far along you were, "It wasn't a baby just yet." I disagree with all of the above. You have a right to grieve, to cry, scream and to take all the time you need to move beyond the pain of your loss. Don't believe the lie that miscarriage is a minor event in a woman's life. It is quite the opposite. It's a major pain – a hole left in your heart that only God can heal.

When it happened to us, I fell into a depth of despair so deep that I would rise every morning with tears in my eyes. But I dared not tell anyone what I was going through and what I was *really* feeling. I appeared to be strong in the weakest moments of my life. I, too, suffered in silence. Why do women choose to suffer without support or encouragement from others? They suffer in silence for several reasons such as embarrassment, disappointment, fear of what others will say or some may even feel guilty, as if the miscarriage was their own fault. It honestly made me feel a little less than a woman because my body was not functioning the way God created it to work. The pain you feel is real and you are not alone. The only thing worse than losing the greatest joy of your life is pretending as if you lost nothing.

When I experienced my first miscarriage, I yearned to find women who felt the same pain as I did. I discovered a few of my close friends had miscarriages but found it interesting that most of them never shared their experiences with others, including their partner. I looked for a spiritual resource to help me to move beyond the excruciating disappointment of our loss. I found a few written by women on the other side of this journey - women who had become mothers. But I could not find any written by women who were still waiting in faith (if they had any left) for God to manifest the deepest desire of their hearts, motherhood.

I am writing this book as a childless woman standing in faith that the God who promised I shall lack nothing (Psalm 23:1), will bless with us with the children we desire. I am using my pain for the purpose of freeing many women whom have doubts or fear if they will ever successfully conceive, carry and birth children. How do you move beyond the painful memories and stand strong in your faith? We will take that journey together in this book. If motherhood is your dream, and you are frustrated in reaching your destination, keep reading!

This book is written for every woman and family that still grieves for babies passed from the womb directly into heaven or women who are struggling to experience the

God will not

command us

to do anything

He has not

equipped

us to do.

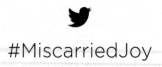

\#MiscarriedJoy

excitement of a positive pregnancy test. There is hope! As we take an inside peek into the lives of women that were once barren in the bible, your faith will be strengthened, you will find a new hope in the God that created life and you will be thoroughly equipped to put on the full armor of God to fight (and win) against the tactics of the enemy. The God who created life has the power and ability to fill your womb and bring forth His child through you at His appointed time. We will dispel the myth that God caused your miscarriage. We will look into the hearts of barren or infertile women and see how their faith carried them into the manifestation of their destiny. As you turn the pages of this book, you may cry, reflect and learn more about the heart of Jesus Christ.

"Then God blessed them and said, "Be fruitful and multiply. Fill the earth and govern it. Reign over the fish in the sea, the birds in the sky, and all the animals that scurry along the ground." (Genesis 1:28)

God will not command us to do anything He has not equipped us to do. God placed the desire to have children in your heart, but the enemy fights against the divine purposes of Christ. If you want to win against the enemy, you must fight in prayer and faith. You can grieve, but at some point you have to get up, get dressed in your armor and firmly believe that God will grant you every desire of your heart. You must shift your focus off of what happened and turn it towards seeking strength from God and trust in His promises.

"For the Lord God is a sun and a safe-covering. The Lord gives favor and honor. He holds back nothing good from those who walk in the way that is right." (Psalm 84:11)

Not everything we want is what God desires for us. He does not promise to give us everything *we* want, but in this verse He promises that He will not withhold what is permanently good for us. He has equipped each of us with the same measure of faith, but we must activate it and exercise it to bring about the manifestation for what we believe God to do in our lives. We are taking the steps to move beyond incredible pain to extraordinary faith. Let's take this journey together!

CHAPTER 1

A Miscarried Secret

"We can't find a heartbeat."
"The fetus did not implant in the uterus."
"The fetus isn't developing properly."

You may have heard these words from an ultrasound technician or from your physician during a routine pre-natal exam. You probably cried many tears, because I sure did. Day after day, I ran into my husband's arms and just cried. We had suffered so great a loss but not many could understand the depth of our heartbreak. After learning of your loss, how did you truly feel and who did you tell? If you are like most women, you probably only exposed your miscarried bundle of joy with a chosen few. Miscarriage is the most common type of pregnancy loss, according to the American College of Obstetricians and Gynecologists (ACOG).

Studies reveal that anywhere from 10-25% of all clinically recognized pregnancies will end in miscarriage.[1] The most common reason for miscarriage stems from chromosomal abnormalities in the fetus. An increase in maternal age can also affect the chances of miscarriage.

- Women under the age of thirty-five years old have about a 15% chance of miscarriage
- Women between the ages of thirty-five and forty-five have a 20 percent to 35 percent chance of miscarriage
- Women over the age of forty-five have a fifty percent chance of miscarriage
- Women who have experienced a previous miscarriage have a 25 percent chance of having another one. (This is only a slight increase than someone who has not had a previous miscarriage)[2]

Pregnancy loss is a very common, yet unspoken event that many women experience. Maurice and I chose not to share it with many people, but it definitely became a major focus of our conversation and prayers with God. It is a loss that touches more women around us than we often realize. When you look at the above statistics, it may shed a bit of light into why many people who have not experienced miscarriage have the opinion that it is not a loss as great as the pain you feel. After our first pregnancy loss, I did extensive research on the causes to see if there was anything I could have done to prevent it. I questioned if it was my fault. Did I exercise too much, not get enough rest, eat or drink the wrong things? I placed the blame on me and for a moment, also on God. I began to search the scriptures to learn about what God said about miscarriage. Here is what I found in the Word of God:

"You must serve only the Lord your God. If you do, I will bless you with food and water, and I will protect

Knowing God is more

sufficient than

knowing the *whys*

of our *sufferings*.

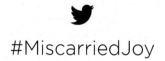

#MiscarriedJoy

you from illness. **There will be no miscarriages or infertility in your land,** *and I will give you long, full lives." (Exodus 23:25-26)*

"In the same way, **it is not my heavenly Father's will that even one of these little ones should perish."** (Matthew 18:14) - God is concerned about every human being that He has created.

"You will experience all these blessings if you obey the Lord your God: Your towns and your fields will be blessed. **Your children and your crops will be blessed.** *The offspring of your herds and flocks will be blessed. Your fruit baskets and breadboards will be blessed. Wherever you go and whatever you do, you will be blessed." (Deuteronomy 28:2-6)*

How could something so common in the world be the opposite of what God has promised to His children? If God promised His children there would be no miscarriages or barrenness in the land, then why has it happened to so many women that serve Him? Is this a contradiction of His Word? How could a God who is so loving take away our heart's greatest joy? Isn't He the God who is faithful to fulfill what He promised? Isn't He the God who will fully equip our bodies to function according to His design?

Having children has proved to be challenging for many women. Some women struggle to conceive or successfully carry a baby to term. In a survey of married women, the CDC found that 1.5 million women in the US (6%) are infertile.[3] It is a great disappointment to desire to have a child and feel there is a possibility you will be unable to be fruitful and multiply. It can be one of the deepest levels of pain for women.

It affects our confidence, potentially shatters our dreams and makes some regret that we haven't *yet* been able to give our husbands the sons or daughters they desire.

It is a wound opened over and over again every time someone asks the dreaded question, "When are you going to have a baby?" I don't know about you, but whenever someone asks me about having a baby, the pain of my losses return, and I mentally and emotionally relive the moments of losing our angel babies. I celebrate those around me birthing their bundles of joy while still dealing with the current reality that the children we desperately desire has proved to be one of the greatest mountains we've ever had to climb. "Lord, when are you going to do this for me?" is a question many childless women bring to the feet of Jesus in their private prayer time.

Did you think conceiving and carrying a baby to term would be easy? I sure did. In fact, I thought it would be easier to get pregnant than it was to prevent it. I never fathomed that starting a family would be one of the most difficult challenges we would encounter in our marriage. I was certain we could time it according to when *we* were ready by using our choice of preventative measures. Then, once we were ready to conceive, it would happen with no challenges, little delays and zero complications. Boy was I wrong! Everything we have experienced has been quite the opposite and you probably feel the same way. I understand the heartbreak that lives with you daily. I know the frustrations of waiting and wondering, asking and doubting, smiling while suffering silently. There aren't enough words in any language that could describe the tremendous amount of tears that you have cried, alone.

Why is it so many struggle with repeated miscarriage and infertility, but it's such a taboo topic to discuss? We don't talk about it with most of our family, our close circle of friends, our pastors, or mentors, and it's certainly not a social media announcement! Instead, behind closed doors we remember. We remember the cold ultrasound room, the tears that left our eyes as the news was delivered, the outline of a baby on the screen with no heartbeat, the missing fetus that never developed, or the repeated pregnancy tests that were all negative. The growing belly, gender reveal and baby shower would not be occurring within the next nine months. We know all too well what it's like to go from cloud nine excitement to the deepest depth of discouragement. The shoulders of our husbands, and maybe our pillows, are the only ones that really know the suffering we are encountering. We wake up in the morning, get dressed, go to work, run businesses, smile and celebrate others while silently, we are suffering. We are crying on the inside while glowing on the outside. We are dealing with death without being able to openly mourn.

Miscarriage is a silent suffering. It's a private matter we dare not discuss publicly. I am choosing to break the silence in hopes that my story will transform the faith of so many women who are still waiting for their children to manifest on this side of heaven. Maybe one day, you will do the same. You are not alone and you should not have to suffer and heal alone.

It is challenging to find women who will openly share the details of their story, their pain, fears, doubts and healing. Speaking out can help so many people. Many women don't share that they have become the mother of an angel for various reasons that are personal to each person. Maybe it's because we are ashamed or we don't want others to know

His wisdom,

justice

and love greatly

overshadows

our suffering.

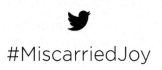

#MiscarriedJoy

we were unsuccessful in our attempts to conceive, carry and birth a child. Maybe it's because we don't want other women to be discouraged in their efforts and hopes of conceiving. Whatever your choice is for not sharing (if that has been your story), you have a right to do what you feel is best for you.

But I pray this book is a step towards all women feeling open enough to share their pain for the purpose of helping other women to heal emotionally and spiritually. Many women wonder why God has allowed their precious bundle of joy to be stripped away from the arms that once would hold their son or daughter. Lord, why? Why did you allow this to happen to us? We serve you, we desperately want children, but we are struggling. We want to multiply but we have been unable to successfully bear the fruit of our offspring. God, what is your purpose in this pain?

YOUR JOB EXPERIENCE

Jesus Christ – the King of all Kings - where is He in this? How is His love being displayed in my loss? Why did He take my babies from me? Is this God's fault? These were the questions I found myself asking plenty of times – even after my second miscarriage. How could my Father who is so loving, so perfect and so sovereign take my babies from me? I was reminded of Job. Just in case you aren't familiar with his story, let me share a little of it with you. Job was a blameless man of complete integrity. He feared God and stayed far away from evil. Job was a very wealthy man with seven sons and three daughters, an abundance of sheep, camels, oxen and donkeys (Job 1). Let's just say Job didn't want for anything and had enough wealth to share for generations to come. He was surely living the abundant life mentioned in John 10:10.

> *One day the members of the heavenly court came to present themselves before the Lord, and the Accuser, Satan, came with them. "Where have you come from?* *The Lord asked Satan. Satan answered the Lord, "I have been patrolling the earth, watching everything that's going on. Then the Lord asked Satan, "Have you noticed my servant Job? He is the finest man in all the earth. He is blameless - a man of complete integrity. He fears God and stays away from evil. Satan replied to the Lord, "Yes, but Job has good reason to fear God. You have always put a wall of protection around him and his home and his property. You have made him prosper in everything he does. Look how rich he is! But reach out and take away everything he has, and he will surely curse you to your face!" "All right,* **you may test him**,*" the Lord said to Satan. "*Do whatever you want with everything he possesses, but don't harm him physically.*" So Satan left the Lord's presence. (Job 1:6-12)*

God was well pleased with Job and His commitment to living his life according to God's commandments. Isn't it both powerful and refreshing to know that God had to give Satan permission to test Job? Satan felt like it made perfect sense in the natural for Job to love God so wholeheartedly because God had allowed him to prosper in everything. Satan was sure that if Job had lost the resources that made his life so comfortable and fulfilling, he would surely turn away from God!

As you read the story of Job in its entirety, calamity breaks out before chapter one even comes to a close. Job's character

God's intention in the

test is to increase and

prove the *strength*

of our character and

the *fortitude*

of our faith.

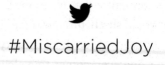

#MiscarriedJoy

is attacked, he loses his property, his children, and then his health deteriorates! I don't know about you, but at this point, I would just about lose it. His own wife told him to curse God and die. But through all of his suffering, Job remained faithful to God. In spite of the great losses that he suffered, he acknowledged God's sovereign authority over everything he possessed. He truly loved God for who he was and not for what He was able to give.

While we are sitting in this season of waiting for children and having our angel babies taken from us, you may, like me, feel like Job in various aspects. Living in a society of instant gratification has negatively impacted our ability to trust God's timing and wait. How do you think Job felt when he lost not one, not two, but all of his children? Job had built a life with his sons and daughters. He loved each one of them from the very depths of his heart, yet God had allowed them to be taken away at the very blink of an eye. Don't you sympathize with Job because you, too, know what it feels like for the child whom you love (before you've ever laid eyes on them) to be snatched? Job asked God why (Job 10:3, 13:23-24) and I am sure you also asked God why he chose you to suffer such an unexplainable pain. I know I did. But *knowing* God is more sufficient than knowing the *whys* of our sufferings.

There have been moments in my life when I felt like Job. I felt as if the deepest desires of my heart were taken from me with no reason why. But here is the truth God wants us to see through our trials of repeated miscarriages and infertility - His wisdom, justice and love *greatly* overshadows our suffering. God is not the cause of your miscarriage or inability to conceive. He allowed you to experience this pain to strengthen your faith, to deepen your relationship with

Him and to create an opportunity for you to see He has His hand on your life in such a way that your coming victory could only be because of Him!

God is the Creator of all things. He is accountable to no one and has authority over all. He is sovereign, The King with the highest status. He rules and reigns over our lives, our desires, our suffering, our challenges and our triumphs. He is the author of our situations. God's stamp of approval is on your story because He already knows the outcome of your situation. We must not have a limited understanding and acceptance of God's wisdom. If we refuse to accept only the good and do away with the bad, we may completely reject what God is trying to do through us when things don't work out the way we desired. God is in control of all things and he permits His children to endure testing. That's right, ladies. This journey we are walking through together is a test.

"Consider it a sheer gift, friends, when tests and challenges come at you from all sides. You know that under pressure, your faith-life is forced into the open and shows its true colors. So don't try to get out of anything prematurely. Let it do its work so you become mature and well-developed, not deficient in any way." (John 1:2-4 MSG)

A gift?! What about this suffering is a gift? I had to spend some time meditating on the above scripture, because wanting a baby and experiencing difficulties having one didn't exactly feel like a box I would joyfully open! The Holy Spirit led me to think about the end result. Imagine unwrapping a box to find just a few puzzle pieces. The images on each piece aren't even enough for you to have some idea

The blessings that come

without *challenges*

sometimes aren't

appreciated

as much as those that

arrive *after* a struggle.

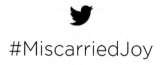

#MiscarriedJoy

of the final picture. Then there is a note at the bottom that says this:

> *"Every day, you will be gifted with a small puzzle piece as you travel along this journey of life. Some pieces will be for your picture and some will be for others. It may be quite a frustrating experience now because your burden has become heavy, but at the end of your journey, you will see the beautiful picture I was creating all along."* Love, God.

Each piece of the puzzle represents each moment we experience in our lives, good or bad. If we continue to trust God is in control, we will see that He was always working all things out for our good. God's intention in allowing us to be tested is to increase and prove the strength of our character and the fortitude of our faith. It is our response to the testing that determines the effect it will have in our lives and in our relationship with Jesus Christ. Though Satan was working against Job, it was God who allowed or authorized everything that was happening in Job's life. God promises us that we will not be tempted beyond what we can endure.

You, woman of God, can endure this. It is only a test of your faith. Will you rise up and pray or will you throw in the towel and give up? Will you allow God to use you to strengthen the faith of other women believing for children or will you, like many, convince yourself that maybe, just maybe, God doesn't hear the cries of your heart? How will your response to this test of faith impact the outcome?

> *"The temptations in your life are no different from what others experience. And God is faithful. He will not allow*

the temptation to be more than you can stand. When you are tempted, he will show you a way out so that you can endure." (1 Corinthians 10:13)

*"No **test or temptation** that comes your way is beyond the course of what others have had to face. All you need to remember is that God will never let you down; **he'll never let you be pushed past your limit;** he'll always be there to help you come through it." (1 Corinthians 10:13 MSG)*

"Hardships often prepare ordinary people for an extraordinary destiny." (C.S. Lewis)

The blessings that come without challenges sometimes aren't appreciated as much as those that arrive after a struggle. Many things in life have come easy to me, including degrees, jobs, good grades, etcetera. I don't say this to boast or brag. I say it because this realization was a vivid revelation for me. The absence of real challenges in my life has not afforded me the opportunity to build my faith in the area of trusting God to do the impossible. I often pray and believe God to work miracles in the lives of others, but when I need a miracle, doubt kicks into gear. I have witnessed God work miracles for others. Since He is not a respecter of persons and doesn't show favoritism, then why wouldn't He manifest what I am confessing?

God is our Father; thus, He corrects, disciplines and rewards us in a similar manner as our earthly father may have done. As we are in this season of testing, awaiting our precious babies from heaven, I am convinced that God is conditioning our faith to trust Him on levels we've never had to before. He wants our test to be evidence of His miracles to encourage others who will eventually walk in these same shoes. He has authorized everything that is happening, or not happening, in our lives. Where is your level of faith and what events or challenges have occurred in your life that have strengthened your faith? If your situation is currently contrary to what you prayed for, will you allow your situation to have authority over you? What will you authorize for your life or will you allow Satan to write the end of this chapter.

The Word has the final authority over your life and God's Word says,

> *"That is why we never give up. Though our bodies are dying, our spirits are being renewed every day. For our present troubles are small and won't last very long. Yet they produce for us a glory that vastly outweighs them and will last forever! So we don't look at the troubles we can see now; rather, we fix our gaze on things that cannot be seen. For the things we see now will soon be gone, but the things we cannot see will last forever." (2 Corinthians 4:16-18)*

Job didn't curse God, He endured.

The children of Israel were delivered and entered into the Promised Land - after enduring plagues.

Paul and Silas didn't give up. They praised their way through and the prison doors were opened.

Daniel wasn't intimated by the lion. His prayers and belief in God shut the mouth of the lion.

Shadrach, Meshach and Abed-Nego didn't die in the fire. Their belief and trust in the God they served faithfully delivered them from the fiery furnace.

The Israelites didn't stop on six. They marched around the seventh time as instructed and Jericho was delivered into their hands.

And you will be delivered from the disappointments you have experienced. The other side of this looks so much greater than the view of your current circumstance. Keep walking through the valley and climbing over the mountain. Don't stop believing God to perform the impossible, improbable and amazing miracle you are waiting on. Just as Job, Daniel and the Israelites endured the test, you, too, must endure. You must pray, praise, worship and trust your way through this situation until your Jericho is delivered unto you! The babies you desire will come. But it requires faith - the faith that is small as a mustard seed, but mighty enough to move mountains. You must endure and overcome the temporary pain and emptiness of your temporary infertility or ability to conceive, carry and birth. You have the power to say "This is not how my story is going to end." And so shall it be.

God had His hand on every test displayed throughout the Bible and these stories are a reminder of God's power from generations past and for generations to come. Your story may not be for you. Maybe it's for someone else. God uses us for His glory and often it doesn't feel good; it's uncomfortable, it's hurtful, disappointing, and maybe even unfair. Your hardship is just a requirement for the manifestation of your destiny! It is an opportunity to build a relationship with God that will be stronger because of what you have experienced.

CHAPTER 2

Pushing Through the Pain

*"Don't let your hearts be troubled. Trust in
God, and trust also in me." (John 14:1)*

*"Yet what we suffer now is nothing compared to the
glory he will reveal to us later." (Romans 8:18)*

Pain. Disappointment. Discouragement. It's an unfortunate reality that every person experiences throughout life. We lose our confidence or enthusiasm towards something we once looked forward to. You know the job you thought you had in the bag but the offer never came through? Did you become discouraged? What about the business deal you were once so sure of that fell through the cracks? Discouraged now? Let's bring it a little closer to home. What about the news of so many women around you having babies with no issues, while *you* are struggling to conceive or carry to term? I don't know about you but I have definitely had some moments at the lowest levels of discouragement one could reach – the level where you just totally give up and find another option. Yes, that has been me. I bet Sarah, Rebekah, Rachel, Elizabeth and Hannah had bouts of discouragement, pain and the desire to just throw in the towel during various pit stops in their journeys to motherhood, too. All of these women have an intimate knowledge of our pain. They were once barren or infertile - unable to birth the fruit of their offspring. Their husbands felt what our husbands feel - wanting to become a father but losing hope when their wives lose babies or fail to see a plus sign on a pregnancy test.

"Hope deferred makes the heart sick, but a dream fulfilled is a tree of life." (Proverbs 13:12)

In biblical times, barrenness was a woman's greatest misfortune. Children were a necessity for the perpetual growth of the family's tribe. The outcome of a woman's infertility could lead to a loss of inheritance, along with social and financial ruin. The perception of women in the bible was that it was their responsibility and sole purpose in life to conceive and birth children. No wonder we feel so much pressure to have children today! It has been passed down from Eve's generation to ours. Children were required to fulfill God's purpose for mankind - to be fruitful and multiply.

"Children are a blessing from the Lord and a reward from Him." (Psalm 127:3).

"When the Lord saw that Leah was unloved, he enabled her to have children, but Rachel could not conceive." (Genesis 29:31)

God's Word reveals and

confronts our sin,

confirms God's *grace*

in our lives, helps us to

realign our *priorities*,

and equips us to live a life

that is *pleasing* to God.

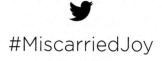

#MiscarriedJoy

God used fertility to reward and comfort both Leah and the Shunammite woman (2 Kings 4:8-17). Yet, He never condemned any woman because of her inability to bear children. So if you are condemning or blaming yourself for your *temporary* infertility, stop doing so now. When God dealt with Israel as a nation in the Old Testament, His blessings were directly related to the strength and wealth of the nation. Children were a metaphor for God's blessings. The pressure to bear children in biblical days and perhaps even now, was more cultural than it was spiritual. Women in those days had so much pressure on them to conceive due to the cultural norms.

Today, that is not the case. The pressure we place on ourselves to have children is still very present and, for some, an unavoidable reality. After God, family is the most important element of our lives. It's one of the ways in which we define ourselves, our past, and how we see ourselves in the context of the world around us. It's where we build our legacies. It's often the place we run to when all hell is breaking loose in our lives. Family is where we receive the love, care, concern and support we need to keep running the race we call life. Family, the people you must live with while also being the people you cannot live without. Those who grew up without the love of a close-knit family often seek it by building their own. It can be a source of pressure we place on ourselves. It's easy to feel lost or have minimal sense of purpose when we don't have a close family or encounter challenges building one of our very own. The concept of family has been extremely important since the beginning of time. It was first introduced in Genesis 1:28. God's plan for the human creation was for men and women to unite as one in marriage and have children; to create families, the fundamental building block of society.

God honored the familial covenant so much that two of the Ten Commandments are centered around the family bond. *"Honor your father and mother. Then you will live a long, full life in the land the Lord your God is giving you" (Exodus 20:12).* This commandment was purposed to protect and preserve the authority that fathers and mothers possess in family matters and over their children.

"You must not commit adultery" (Exodus 20:14). This commandment prohibits infidelity and thus proves that God's heart is to protect the sanctity of marriage. The strength and health of family was so important to God that He placed commandments that all of His children must obey. Family is not an Old Testament tradition. The New Testament reemphasizes the family covenant. Jesus also speaks about the sanctity of marriage and how he hates divorce in Matthew 19. The apostle Paul gives an image of what Christian homes should mirror in Ephesians 6:1-4.

> *"Children, obey your parents because you belong to the Lord, for this is the right thing to do. "Honor your father and mother." This is the first commandment with a promise: If you honor your father and mother, "things will go well for you, and you will have a long life on the earth." Fathers, do not provoke your children to anger by the way you treat them. Rather, bring them up with the discipline and instruction that comes from the Lord."*

Obeying these commands rewards you with the promise of long life on the earth. Yes, family is just that important. Today, we want to give our children what our parents gave us, or maybe what they were unable to provide. We want the opportunity to raise another generation of men and women who would make our parents proud. We want to extend the love that was placed in our hearts within our own homes, being prayerful that it extends out into the world around us. Who wouldn't want to have a sense of belonging in the earth? What better place than our own homes, with our families, the ones that we've continued to build for generation to generation?

Our desire to have children is so strong that when we discover the challenges, we allow discouragement to settle in our minds and hearts. God didn't bless Hannah with Samuel simply because he felt compassion for her discouragement. He blessed Hannah because she cried out of a place of extraordinary faith. Sarah was certainly discouraged along her journey to motherhood. She was ninety years old when she and Abraham received the prophecy that they would be blessed with a son! There are other women in the bible, who we will discuss in depth in the chapters to come, who did not allow their disappointment and discouragement to permanently keep them from the promise.

Discouragement is often the emotional response to the sufferings we experience in our lives. It is normal but we must be careful to not allow this debilitating emotion to get the very best of us. You and I are not the only ones who have felt like giving up. Our family and friends may not know what to say to us, simply because they don't understand the pain and disappointment we feel in this journey. Job felt discouraged by his family and friends for the same reason. They just didn't get it! Our fervent prayers to God aren't always answered in the way we desire. Elijah knows that feeling well.

He became discouraged when his ministry didn't produce the results he had hoped for (1 Kings 19). Peter took his focus off God while walking on the water and began to sink

Discouragement leads to

doubt and *unbelief,*

and temporarily *blinds*

us to the truths and power

that *Christ* possesses.

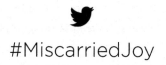

#MiscarriedJoy

(Matthew 14:22-31). That's what really happens when we allow discouragement to settle into our hearts and minds - we take our focus off the power of God and begin to hone in on our circumstances. The danger of discouragement is allowing it to linger for too long; then we consider quitting on the dream or desires in our hearts. But if we give up where we are, we will never receive the manifestation of the promises from God.

"That is why we never give up. Though our bodies are dying, our spirits are being renewed every day. For our present troubles are small and won't last very long. Yet they produce for us a glory that vastly outweighs them and will last forever! So we don't look at the troubles we can see now; rather, we fix our gaze on things that cannot be seen. For the things we see now will soon be gone, but the things we cannot see will last forever." (2 Corinthians 4:16-18)

Discouragement happens to the best of us. But how do we conquer it – especially when our circumstance remains the same? I am not the author who is going to tell you *to* do something without equipping you with the necessary tools to carry it out. My husband and I have been trying to have a baby for almost two years and, while that might not seem like a long time to some, it is the most difficult thing I have ever had to endure. I often cry in secret after hearing my husband say "I can't wait to have a son!" I want to give him a son just as bad as he wants one, if not more. In my life, I have always been able to have control and easily access the things I wanted. This is a situation that is totally in God's control.

After losing three babies, I am so anxious for another positive pregnancy test, yet a bit fearful that what has already happened could happen again. Yes, I know, fear not, be anxious for nothing and have faith. But we are being honest here. There have been moments when it's been downright difficult to walk in faith. Many days and nights I have cried out to God asking Him to strengthen my faith, remove my fears and help me to hold fast to my confession of faith. I asked, "God, how do I overcome this discouragement to focus on Your Word and to get to the other side of this mountain?" How in the world do I overcome this when my situation remains unchanged?

FACING DISCOURAGEMENT

"But I, the Lord, search all hearts and examine secret motives. I give all people their due rewards, according to what their actions deserve." (Jeremiah 17:10)

The first step to overcoming discouragement is to be totally honest and transparent with God. He knows our hearts and every thought that enters our minds. It won't do you any good to pretend that your anger, frustration, disappointment or fears don't exist. Tell God about every single feeling you have and ask Him to heal your hurts, fill your voids, erase your fears and help you to rest in knowing that His plan is perfect and so is His timing. I don't like waiting, but in this I have no choice. When I emptied my heart to God, he began to strengthen my faith in Him day by day. God allowed me to see my trial as a source of joy and an opportunity to know Him in a way that I have never known Him before. I am reminded of the encouragement that James gives when he says,

"My brethren, count it all joy when you fall into various trials, knowing that the testing of your faith produces patience. But let patience have its perfect work, that you may be perfect and complete, lacking nothing." (James 1:2-4 NKJV)

Troubles in life are inevitable. Your decisions drive the outcome of your circumstance. You don't have to pretend to be happy, but you do need to have a positive outlook on the situation. You may not have a baby *yet*, but you will. You may have had to experience loss, but soon you will experience great gains. Troubles can produce a lot in our lives, but only if we persevere in the face of opposition. Ask God what He wants you to learn from this situation you are facing. Ask Him how He wants to use your story for His glory.

I, like you, am still waiting on the babies I know God promised me. But while I am in waiting, I am using my pain for a purpose - to encourage you. The depth of our character is revealed by how we respond under pressure. It's easy to be cheerful when all is going well, but will we still trust God when life just doesn't seem fair? We overcome discouragement by the power and truth of God's Word.

The Word of God brings an immense amount of comfort and reassurance. The thing that will refresh you the most in the midst of feeling discouraged is to hear God speaking to your specific circumstances through His Word. Search the scriptures to see what God says about the emotions you are experiencing, the pain that you feel and the joy that may be missing. Even when you don't feel like reading His word, go against your feelings.

"God means what he says. What he says goes. His powerful Word is sharp as a surgeon's scalpel, cutting through everything, whether doubt or defense, laying us open to listen and obey. Nothing and no one is impervious to God's Word. We can't get away from it – no matter what." (Hebrews 4:12-13 MSG)

God's Word serves multiple purposes in our lives. The Word reveals and confronts our sin, confirms God's grace in our lives, helps us to realign our priorities, and equips us to live a life that is pleasing to God. *"In the beginning was the Word, and the Word was with God, and the Word was God"* (John 1:1). God and His Word are one and the same. It's the Word of God that washes out every impurity, negative thought, ungodly emotion, fear, anxiety and anything else that keeps you from living life as God has purposed you to live. Stay intimately connected to the vine, especially through the circumstances that make it easy to run away from God.

"I am the true grapevine, and my Father is the gardener. He cuts off every branch of mine that doesn't produce fruit, and he prunes the branches that do bear fruit so they will produce even more. You have already been pruned and purified by the message I have given you. Remain in me, and I will remain in you. For a branch cannot produce fruit if it is severed from the vine, and you cannot be fruitful unless you remain in me. "Yes, I am the vine; you are the branches. Those who remain in me, and I in them, will produce much fruit. For apart from me you can do nothing. Anyone who does not remain in me is thrown away like a useless branch and withers. Such branches are gathered into a pile to be burned. But if you

remain in me and my words remain in you, you may ask for anything you want, and it will be granted! When you produce much fruit, you are my true disciples. This brings great glory to my Father. (John 15:1-6)

Another major function of God's Word is to realign our thinking to God's thinking. Through His Word, the Holy Spirit continually conforms our minds to focus on how God operates. Rather than thinking about what seems impossible, you will begin to concentrate on God performing the impossible in your life. We must learn to have the right view of God in order to overcome the discouragement that happens when our fervent prayers aren't answered. Yes, God can work beyond your age being past "child-bearing" years, your fears of not being able to successfully carry to term or any other cause of infertility. If you think God can't, then He won't. The bible is God's tools to renew your mind concerning your life and your situation.

"But it was to us that God revealed these things by his Spirit. For his Spirit searches out everything and shows us God's deep secrets. No one can know a person's thoughts except that person's own spirit, and no one can know God's thoughts except God's own Spirit. And we have received God's Spirit (not the world's spirit), so we can know the wonderful things God has freely given us." (1 Corinthians 2:10-12)

God is above all and everything is under His control. In times of suffering, it is helpful to search His Word to be reminded of who He really is in our lives and the power He has to turn around every challenge we encounter.

Doubting God

confirms that

you have little

faith in Him.

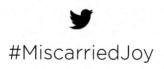

#MiscarriedJoy

"God sits above the circle of the earth. The people below seem like grasshoppers to him! He spreads out the heavens like a curtain and makes his tent from them. "To whom will you compare me? Who is my equal?" asks the Holy One. Look up into the heavens. Who created all the stars? He brings them out like an army, one after another, calling each by its name. Because of his great power and incomparable strength, not a single one is missing. O Jacob, how can you say the Lord does not see your troubles? O Israel, how can you say God ignores your rights? Have you never heard? Have you never understood? The Lord is the everlasting God, the Creator of all the earth. He never grows weak or weary. No one can measure the depths of his understanding." (Isaiah 40:21, 25-28)

There is strength in the Word of God. *"Therefore my dears [sisters], stand firm. Let nothing move you. Always give yourselves fully to the work of the Lord, because you know that your labor (pain, anguish or suffering) in the Lord is not in vain" (1 Corinthians 15:58 NIV).* Having a depth of knowledge of the Scriptures affects our mindsets toward our present sufferings and our future conditions. The more we are reminded about what God has done in the lives of others, the more confidence we have about what He is capable of doing in our lives. If you want to overcome discouragement, dive into the Word, which is meant to encourage you.

"I want them to be encouraged and knit together by strong ties of love. I want them to have complete confidence that they understand God's mysterious plan, which is Christ himself. In him lie hidden all the treasures of wisdom and knowledge." (Colossians 2:2)

Being discouraged is a trick of the enemy. If Satan can keep our minds focused on what God has not done, we won't focus on our faith or stand firm on what we are asking God to do. A miracle won't happen in our future if we are still concerned about our present circumstances. God's word reveals His character and his heart. The scriptures reveal God to be holy, loving, just, gracious, eternal, merciful and infinitely good. A Father like that does not desire for you to live in a sea of discouragement. It is in His Word where He reveals His power in impossible situations. Jesus fed five-thousand men plus women and children with two fish and five loaves of bread (John 6:1-14). That's the kind of provision He freely gives. He walked on water to rescue His disciples (Matthew 14:22-33). That's the kind of care and concern that He extends. He raised Lazarus from the dead (John 11). That is the healing power He exhibits. The great news is this - the same things that Christ has done for others, He can surely do for you and me.

"Even Elizabeth your relative is going to have a child in her old age, and she who was said to be barren is in her sixth month. For nothing is impossible with God." (Luke 1:36-37)

CONQUERING DISCOURAGEMENT

So what do you do when this dangerous emotion seems like you can't just fight it off? First, you must realize it's a decision you make. You don't have to be discouraged, you choose to be. Through the power of Christ, you are equipped to handle every situation you are faced with. The Holy Spirit is your helper. You have The Word of God and the amazing privilege of prayer to assist you in conquering this emotion which comes from the enemy. Tell Satan that he will not have your joy or your peace. You must also maintain the right attitude. What we allow to take residence in our minds is what will come out in our actions and our words. If you think you are discouraged, you will continually speak it and are at risk of discouraging others as well.

> *"Sisters, whatever is true, whatever is noble, whatever is right, whatever is pure, whatever is lovely, whatever is admirable – if anything is excellent or praiseworthy – think about such things." (Philippians 4:8)*

Ask God to help you focus on the blessings He has brought into your life. Let's not focus on this one thing and risk being happy about what God is still doing. You are still healthy and whole. Our babies are coming!

Surround yourself with people who will encourage you and pray for you. I know it's tough to reveal the pain of miscarriages, stillbirths or infertility. But ask God to show you at least one person who can unite with you in prayer and join their faith with yours. It is a true blessing when you have a praying woman on your side who can ease your doubts when they creep in and remind you that God hears your cries. I think Renee Swope put it best when she said, *"Asking for prayer isn't about putting burdens on friends. It's about letting them walk with us down a path that you were never meant to walk alone."* God places people in our lives for a purpose. Your true friends will want to experience the greatest moments in your life and be there for you through your greatest disappointments. Allow them that privilege. God blessed you with them because he knew you would need them for times such as these.

Be a blessing to others! Encourage and celebrate others who are experiencing the joy you still stand in faith to receive. That's what I do. I chose to rejoice with those who rejoice (Romans 12:15) and shifted my focus on the amazing women in my circle who are having babies. I committed to sowing into those women. I sowed happiness, love, encouraging words, prayers, tears of joy and gifts. I was in the midst of planning a baby shower for my cousin when I found out my third baby didn't have a heartbeat. I could have wallowed in sadness but I didn't. I went shopping for cupcakes and cake pops with babies on them. I purchased balloons and decorated her shower to bring the brightest smile to her face - all while I was dying on the inside. I ensured that she had an amazing day filled with love and not once did I mention what was happening with me.

Why? Because this was her time and although I couldn't see it at that moment, I knew my time would come. I had people ask me was this hard to do. It wasn't, because my love and happiness for her would not allow my loss to dim her light. That is the place where God wants us to be. He wants us to celebrate the blessings of others regardless of what we are experiencing. It helps you to slap discouragement in the face, conquer your fears, and erase your doubts. The Word of God promises that where we sow, we will reap (Galatians 6:7, Luke 6:38). After my miscarriages, I sent a gift to every baby shower I was invited to even if I was unable to make it. I am expecting to one day soon have my own baby shower and thus, I am sowing into the lives of those that God is blessing; I am not jealous in the least bit. I am ecstatic because every *"We are expecting"* news is a reminder of what God can do.

The *depth* of our

character is *revealed*

by how we *respond*

under pressure.

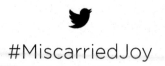

#MiscarriedJoy

The Dangers of Discouragement

The pain you feel about not yet being able to conceive, carry or birth a child is deep and real. If you have lost babies on your journey to motherhood, there will always be a special place in your heart where your baby (or babies, for some) reside. You will never forget the moments of happiness nor the moments of misery. But what you can't do is allow the discouragement to take your eyes off of the promise. You have to stand firm in your faith and be cautious in what you release into the atmosphere through thoughts and words. There are hidden dangers that arise when we wallow in the river of discouragement rather than moving on to the ocean of faith.

> *"When you face a difficulty, something you don't understand, instead of being discouraged, instead of complaining, have a new perspective. Declare, "This is not here to defeat me. This is here to promote me." (~ Joel Osteen)*

Discouragement leads to doubt and unbelief, and temporarily blinds us to the truths and power that Christ possesses. Doubting God confirms you have little faith in Him. It also causes you to lose sight of His sovereignty, generosity and love. Faith cannot reside with doubt and be effective. *"But when you ask him, be sure that your faith is in God alone. Do not waver, for a person with divided loyalty is as unsettled as a wave of the sea that is blown and tossed by the wind. Such people should not expect to receive anything from the Lord" (James 1:6).* We must have confidence in God that He will perfectly align our desires with His.

Our temporary circumstance of empty arms is, by faith, just that - *temporary*. We don't have time to reside in our discouragement because it can lead to distractions. Rather than applying our faith and believing God for a miracle, we can easily become tempted to give up or take matters into our own hands. Sarah displayed a lack of faith, trust and patience when she told her husband to sleep with Hagar. I am sure none of us would take such extreme measures as she did, but even small things can signal to God that we don't believe He will do what we have prayed to receive.

Being in a place of discouragement can also lead to carelessness with our words and confessions. What you say has the power to improve or worsen your condition. What you say flows from what is in your heart (Luke 6:45). A heart that is consumed with circumstances is a heart that can easily be hardened - which then leads to anger and resentment towards God. You will begin to think His promises are empty because your arms are too. God has not forgotten about you and the children you desire; the children you think about, dream of, pray for and look forward to having. God will make your dream a reality through your faith and belief in His power to perform. Discouragement has the tendency to make you want to give up and throw in the towel. It can totally zap your energy.

A discouraged woman is dangerous. As women, we should uplift, encourage, edify and equip others to live at their true potential. It's difficult for us to do so effectively when we allow ourselves to remain discouraged for longer than we should. Someone who is discouraged can easily discourage others through negative attitudes and a pessimistic outlook. Rather than speaking words of affirmation, joy and comfort, they tend to leave those in their circle disheartened because they haven't dealt with the pain from their circumstances. If you are walking in faith and confessing your desire to become a mother before God, you cannot afford to allow discouragement to take over your life. Yes, given what we have been through, we have the human right to be disappointed, but the moment discouragement begins to creep into our hearts, we must fight against it. We must get spiritually armed and fight the good fight of faith to conquer discouragement from settling into our minds and hearts. Doubt follows discouragement. The woman who doubts is like a wave of the sea, blown and tossed by the wind and should not expect to receive anything from God (James 1:6 NIV). You must believe!

Part Two:

Faith-Building Lessons from Barren Women

CHAPTER 3

A Premature Birth

Sarah – you probably know a bit about her from your knowledge of the Bible. She was the wife of Abraham, a woman with strong faith, a portrait of true submission. She embodied a gentle and quiet spirit. She was Abraham's ride or die chick. When he came home and told her to pack her bags to travel to a place that he knew nothing about, she got up and did as requested (Genesis 12). I don't know about you but I would be asking some questions! "Abe, where are we going? Why are we going there? Are you sure you heard this from God?" Nope, not Sarah. She just went. Now that is submission and trust in action without doubt or question. She knew Abraham was submitted to and heard from God. She had a unique devotion to her husband. She shared his heartaches and frustrations along with his dreams and blessings. She stood by him through his good choices, bad decisions and challenges. She was an admirable example of a woman who loved unconditionally and persistently. Abraham was promised that he would become the father of many nations, which meant Sarah would become the mother of many nations. But there was a huge issue - Sarah was barren!

Can you imagine your husband coming home with such a great promise God revealed to him – the promise that the two of you will birth not just one nation but *many* nations? I surely would experience pure joy and excitement from the news. But just as Sarah did, I too would question how it would happen at any age beyond fifty! That's exactly when the disappointment would settle it. We know it well - the pain and agony of waiting and waiting and *still* waiting on God's promise to come to pass. I can hear Sarah crying out to God saying, "Lord, I know my husband loves you and communicates with you regularly. But maybe, just maybe, he was confused about your promise because it's been years and I am still waiting. In fact, I am about to take actions into my own hands so my husband can have a child." We know what it feels like to trust in God but have yet to see the manifestation of what we are believing Him to do. We are quite familiar with the tugs on the heartstrings when our husbands mention becoming a father. Isn't it good to know we have someone in the bible who felt this way too? There truly is nothing new under the sun.

"What has been will be again, what has been done will be done again; there is nothing new under the sun." (Ecclesiastes 1:9 NIV)

Together, Abraham and Sarah were asked to firmly believe that God would bless them with a son. They responded with a pure heart of faith, obedience and a promise to tightly

The seed of the

promise requires you to

plant seeds of faith,

trust, *patience* and

long-suffering.

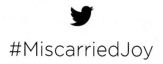

#MiscarriedJoy

hold onto. In the face of famine, they were faithful (Genesis 12). When you decide to follow God's direction, you may encounter great obstacles. Why? Because the enemy doesn't want you to be in God's perfect will because he knows the amazing blessings that will be birthed as a result of your faith. Abraham and Sarah were powerful but they weren't perfect. They acted out of fear a few times in their journey, rather than walking totally in faith. They were human just like you and I. Abraham traveled with Lot (although he was told to leave everything) maybe because he wanted a sense of familiarity and comfort. Later on, they went to Egypt without consulting God when they were faced with famine after leaving their homeland. After years of trying to conceive, they remained unsuccessful.

Abraham and Sarah were experiencing a crisis, at least in Sarah's mind. She had no child! This was a troublesome situation and a source of deep personal pain. As mentioned before, barrenness in 2000 B.C. was a big deal. Today, a childless home is not out of the norm. God promised Abraham that he would be the father of many nations when he was 75 years old. Still, at the age of 85, the promise had not manifested. Sarah's barrenness was not a recent occurrence. What made her condition more painful was that she had a promise without any sign of the manifestation. To begin a great nation, she needed some children! Like you and I, Sarah deeply yearned to hold *her* baby in her arms. She became weary and devised her own plan. Sarah gave her maidservant, Hagar, to lay with Abraham. Ishmael was born. Her impatience led her astray from the perfect will of God. Little did she know, she was still going *through* the necessary process that would transform her into the nurturing woman she would become. Her infertility caused deep humiliation and marital dissension.

For thirteen years, Abraham lived life believing that Ishmael was the manifestation of God's promise to make him the father of many nations. In Genesis 17, in spite of him having a child out of wedlock, God made an unconditional and firm covenant (a definite promise or blessing without conditions) with Abraham. Abraham confirmed the covenant through his obedience to God.

"When Abram was ninety-nine years old, the Lord appeared to him and said, "I am El-Shaddai – 'God Almighty.' Serve me faithfully and live a blameless life. I will make a covenant with you, by which I will guarantee to give you countless descendants." At this, Abram fell face down on the ground. Then God said to him," This is my covenant with you: I will make you the father of a multitude of nations! What's more, I am changing your name. It will no longer be Abram. Instead, you will be called Abraham, for you will be the father of many nations. I will make you extremely fruitful. Your descendants will become many nations, and kings will be among them. "I will confirm my covenant with you and your descendant after you, from generation to generation. This is the everlasting covenant: I will always be your God and the God of your descendants after you. And I will give the entire land of Canaan, where you now live as a foreigner, to you and your descendants. It will be their possession forever, and I will be their God." (Genesis 17:1-8)

God informed Abraham that his blessing of an heir would be manifested through his wife, Sarah. *"Then Abraham bowed down to the ground, but he laughed to himself in disbelief. 'How could I become a father at the age of 100?' he thought. 'And how can Sarah have a baby when she is ninety years old?" (Genesis 17:17).* Sarah still doubted she could become pregnant in her old age. At first she laughed, but eventually reactivated her faith, and believed God would do exactly what He promised her and her husband.

> *"Then one of them said, "I will return to you about this time next year, and your wife, Sarah, will have a son! Sarah was listening to this conversation from the tent. Abraham and Sarah were both very old by this time, and Sarah was long past the age of having children. So she laughed silently to herself and said, "How could a worn-out woman like me enjoy such pleasure, especially when my master – my husband – is also so old?" (Genesis 18:10-12)*

Abraham and Sarah had an abundance of wealth and love. Yet, they remained unfulfilled. Do you feel this way sometimes? Do you have moments when you tend to focus on the fact that God hasn't blessed you with the gift of motherhood, rather than focusing on all He has provided for you? What about all of the ways in which He has protected you? As I deeply reflect on Sarah's actions to "help God out," in addition to her momentary lack of faith, it was her frustration and pain which led her to give Abraham a son in a way that was out of line with God's perfect plan. Even though Sarah fell into sin, God remained faithful in keeping His promise that she would become the "mother of nations" (Genesis 17:16).

"Let us not become weary in doing good, for at the proper time we will reap a harvest if we do not give up." (Galatians 6:9 NIV)

Isn't it easy to become weary even though you are commanded not to? I know it can be a bit discouraging to keep believing and standing firm without any tangible results or rewards. But we can vividly see where impatience lands us from the mistakes that Sarah made. Neglecting to trust God's perfect plan and timing births Ishmaels - seeds of the flesh - in our lives. The seed of the promise is always greater than anything we can produce on our own. I have read the story of Abraham, Sarah, Ishmael and Isaac so many times. But it has given me such a different perspective while waiting for God to manifest the Isaacs in my life. Of course I am not going to find a Hagar and let her lay with my husband to give him a child, but there have been things that we have tried to move our plan of having children very soon right along.

We have purchased ovulation kits, I have tracked my basal body temperature (BBT) and we had intercourse on all the days where I could be ovulating. Still, no positive pregnancy tests. Do you know what it taught me? God is in total control of this! I can't rush the process. I can't force a pregnancy. I can't create life. Only God has the power to do that. He chooses when His promised children will enter this earth and not a moment before. Does it cause weariness to enter my mind? Absolutely! Have I had moments where I have questioned or even doubted God? You bet. What I learned from Sarah is that even though you can try to make things happen on your own, you must surrender to God's plan to bring forth His promise. *"Be still and know that I am God" (Psalm 46:10).*

What is a promise? The Greek word for promise is *"epangelia."* It is an undertaking to give something, a gift graciously bestowed, a gift not secured by a pledge or negotiation; it is conditional upon faith, not upon fulfillment of the law.[4] The Merriam-Webster dictionary defines promise as a declaration or assurance that one will do a particular thing. God is a promise keeper and He will not withhold any good thing from those that walk in obedience to His Word (Psalm 84:11). A promise creates a good ground for expectation. We must wait in great expectation for our children to be conceived and birthed. You must truly believe that despite your age, your condition, your complications, your doctor's reports and your doubts, God will provide the deepest desires of your heart. He will make good on His promises.

Within the union of marriage, it is God's will for you to conceive and birth children. *"He gives the childless woman a family making her a happy mother" (Psalm 113:9).* Scripture teaches that children are a reward from The Lord.

"Children are a gift from the Lord; they are a reward from him. Children born to a young man are like arrows in a warrior's hands. How joyful is the man whose quiver is full of them! He will not be put to shame when he confronts his accusers at the city gates." (Psalm 127:3-5)

The seed of the promise is going to require something of you. It will require you to plant seeds of faith, trust, patience and long-suffering. It will require very close intimacy and time spent with God. You have to become rooted and develop a firm foundation in Christ. We must not place time limits on God. He knew the exact day and time you would be born; thus, it is the same with our children. Their

United faith has

the *power* to birth

what you *believe* God

to do in *your* life.

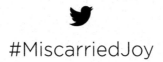

#MiscarriedJoy

purpose is already defined. Their calling has been placed in their hearts and our love for them has already developed. They are our children in the spirit and it *shall* manifest here on earth. It is vital to maintain the eyes of faith in the midst of realizing the fullness of God's perfect promises over your life and your situation. There are many lessons we can learn from the life and legacy of Abraham and Sarah – powerful tools which can be applied in our journeys towards motherhood.

PARTNER IN FAITH

Sarah and Abraham were a trusting couple. They trusted in one another and, more importantly, they trusted God, the One who would lead them to an unknown land with unknown people and unknown situations. Yet, they remained fully confident they would see God's goodness at work in every area of their lives. Even through the laughter, doubt, and faltering of her faith, Sarah trusted God. Abraham and Sarah were a power couple – their partnership in faith led them to become the father and mother in many nations.

God responds to faith! *"By faith we understand that the universe was formed at God's command, so that what is seen was not made out what was visible" (Hebrews 11:3 NIV)*. Faith is the currency of The Kingdom. You must have the Kingdom mindset to get the full benefits, the commonwealth of the Kingdom. Your purpose and ability is locked up in your faith. Everything you want or need is not accessible through your talents or ability, but through the faith (your belief and reliance on the Word of God) you have in Jesus Christ. *"And without faith it is impossible to please God, because anyone who comes to Him must believe that he exists and that he rewards those who earnestly seek him" (Hebrews 11:6).* By faith, Abraham left his home, his comfort zone, to live in a place he did not know. He had no other choice but to be led by God. By faith he made his home in the Promised Land just as a stranger in a foreign land.

"By faith Abraham, even though he was past age – and Sarah herself was barren – was enabled to become a father because he considered him faithful who had made the promise." (Hebrews 11:11)

Though God spoke to Abraham first, he came home to inform Sarah of the instructions he received from God, which would be the guidance to their prayers. Abraham and Sarah became partners, not just in marriage, but in faith. They joined their faith with one another's to stand firm on their belief that God would keep His promises to them. I imagine they too wanted to quit.

"For where two or three gather together as my followers, I am there among them." (Matthew 18:20)

The superficial agreement of thousands will never be as powerful as the heartfelt agreement of a husband and wife in prayer. Why? Because the Holy Spirit is present with them. *"This is the confidence we have in approaching God: that if we ask anything according to his will, he hears us. And if we know that he hears us – whatever we ask – we know that we have what we asked of him (1 John 5:14-15).* Your children are not a blessing for you alone. Your husband has the same desire. So why wouldn't you collaborate in prayer and faith? As I studied what God says about marriage, I found something very interesting – Adam and Jesus had a similar experience before receiving their bride.

Adam was put to sleep before Eve was revealed to him. Jesus was laid in a tomb before He received his bride – the church. Marriage is a perfect reflection of the love Christ has for us. It is a union that requires you to die to yourself. When you get married, you commit to laying down everything pertaining to your old lifestyle of separate goals and plans to be joined to one another. You are much stronger together in prayer than apart!

"How could one chase a thousand, and two put ten thousand to flight, unless their Rock had sold them, And the LORD had surrendered them?." (Deuteronomy 32:30)

When you became united in marriage, your issues became his and vice versa. Your hearts are grafted together, making them dependent on one another for life. The desires you have individually flow into the purpose that is yours collectively. You must believe God for your children together. If you are praying alone and the two of you are not coming together in prayer daily, start now. When your husband is connected to Christ, he hears God and can encourage you in your moments of discouragement. In Genesis 18:9-14, we see God encouraging Sarah through Abraham:

"Where is Sarah, your wife?" the visitors asked.

"She's inside the tent," Abraham replied.

Then one of them said, "I will return to you about this time next year, and your wife, Sarah, will have a son!"

Sarah was listening to this conversation from the tent. Abraham and Sarah were both very old by this time, and Sarah was long past the age of having children. So she laughed silently to herself and said, "How could a worn-

*out woman like me enjoy such pleasure, especially when
my master – my husband – is also so old?"*

*Then the LORD said to Abraham, "Why did Sarah laugh?
Why did she say, 'Can an old woman like me have a
baby?' Is anything too hard for the LORD? I will return
about this time next year, and Sarah will have a son."*

What a powerful display of the oil flowing from the head
in your household! God may speak to your husband about
anything concerning you. This is why is it so pertinent that
you and your husband be united in faith as you pray for
God's promise for your children to come to pass in your life.
We talked to a couple that is dear to our hearts about the
challenges we were experiencing. They shared that God had
them wait for six years to have the son they were praying for.
They were praying and believing together, but they took their
faith to the next level. They went out and bought baby clothes!
The wife hung them up in what would be the nursery. Daily,
they went into *that* closet and thanked God for the son who
would be conceived and birthed very soon. It was shortly after
this act of faith that the manifestation was birthed in their
lives. United faith has the power to birth what you believe
God to do in your life.

Maurice and I wrote a confession for our children that
we speak over our lives daily. I'll share it in another chapter.
There are definitely days when I cry through it because the
trying hasn't yet resulted in success. There are days when I
don't confess it because I allow the enemy to tell me that God
has already heard me and doesn't need to be reminded. But
don't persistent prayers get the attention of heaven? In Luke
18, Jesus tells the parable about the persistent widow:

There is a season of

preparation

we must walk through

for every *blessing*

we receive in our lives.

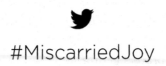

#MiscarriedJoy

One day Jesus told his disciples a story to show that they should always pray and never give up. "There was a judge in a certain city," he said, "who neither feared God nor cared about people. A widow of that city came to him repeatedly, saying, 'Give me justice in this dispute with my enemy.' The judge ignored her for a while, but finally he said to himself, 'I don't fear God or care about people, but this woman is driving me crazy. I'm going to see that she gets justice, because she is wearing me out with her constant requests!'"

Then the Lord said, "Learn a lesson from this unjust judge. Even he rendered a just decision in the end. So don't you think God will surely give justice to his chosen people who cry out to him day and night? Will he keep putting them off? I tell you, he will grant justice to them quickly! But when the Son of Man returns, how many will he find on the earth who have faith?" (Luke 18:1-8)

This woman was persistent. She kept asking the judge until her request was granted. I know that if a judge who doesn't even fear God or care about people will give the woman what she wanted, then my God will definitely grant the deepest desires of my heart as well. So each day, we must confess that the children we desire to love, nurture and raise according to God's Word will be birthed in the physical as long as we war for them in the spiritual. We must not only have faith for today, but faith for eternity. Our faith for today will always be tested and that's why Jesus taught His disciples the principle of persistent prayer.

You may be asking, "Why hasn't God answered my prayer for children yet?" Maybe he hasn't answered your prayers because He is waiting on your continuous prayers before He gives you the ultimate answer. God is both honored and pleased when you remain steadfast in prayer. Jesus said, *"Ask, and it will be given to you; seek, and you will find; knock, and the door will be opened to you"* (Matthew 7:7). How bad do you want children? Keep asking until your arms are no longer empty. Our Father never gets tired of hearing from His children. In fact, He probably doesn't hear from us enough.

OBEDIENCE TO HIS LEADING AND INSTRUCTIONS

"Study this Book of Instruction continually. Meditate on it day and night so you will be sure to obey everything written in it. Only then will you prosper and succeed in all you do. This is my command – be strong and courageous! Do not be afraid or discouraged. For the LORD your God is with you wherever you go." (Joshua 1:8)

In the natural world, prosperity and success come from having power, authority, influence, the ability to strategically network, education and an insistent desire to be successful. When many people think of success, they relate it back to careers, money and business. But I think about success in totality – my career, business, family and pursuing the calling that God has placed on my life. The strategy God taught Joshua for gaining success in the verse above has nothing to do with the world's requirements for success. God tells Joshua that he must obey God's law. Obedience can only be achieved by meditating on God's Word day and night. You cannot obey what you don't know.

I have read Joshua 1:8 many times, but as I was doing research for this book, verse 9 really stood out to me. God commanded that we be strong and courageous. He said not to fear nor be discouraged. God would only tell us this if He knew that in the journey ahead, we would encounter some storms, need to climb some high mountains, swim deep valleys and cross some swinging bridges. God knew every challenge we would encounter in our lives. But the greatest promise is that He is with you wherever you go! The key to any success we want to achieve in your life is obedience. When we give God obedience, He grants us with prosperity and success in every area. It is vital to have full confidence in God's ability and His integrity to fulfill every promise He made in His Word.

Abraham and Sarah's hope was based on the promise of God. Faith is not a passion for what is possible; rather, a requirement for the promised. God terminated twenty-five years of barrenness in Sarah because of her and Abraham's obedience to his instruction for their lives. God can do anything! Your medical diagnosis is of no concern to God. Your age may be a barrier in the natural but definitely not in the spiritual. God has promised to reverse infertility challenges to those that serve and obey Him.

"He gives the childless woman a family, making her a happy mother." (Psalm 113:9)

Disobedience is a refusal to do what God commands in His Word or neglecting to follow the instructions He has given to you for *your* life. Disobedience is very consequential in nature and could end up costing more than you ever imagined. For Sarah, her disobedience occurred when she decided to offer Hagar to Abraham because she grew tired of waiting.

God promised *her* that she, not her maidservant, would give birth to a son. She essentially rejected God's plan and devised her own. This was a very costly mistake. She lost her sense of peace when Hagar began to treat her with contempt. This caused Sarah to mistreat Hagar, probably in hopes she would run away, and that eventually happened. Abraham disobeyed when he heeded the voice of Sarah instead of the voice of God (Genesis 16:2).

There are various consequences to disobedience and God has shown us the cost throughout scripture. Adam and Eve's disobedience of eating the fruit from the Tree of the Knowledge of Good and Evil separated them from the presence of God, brought about toil for men and painful childbirth for women. Moses led the Israelites on a journey to the Promised Land for forty years, but because of his disobedience, he was not able to enter and reap the rewards of the land flowing with milk and honey. Jonah, a prophet of God, was instructed to go to Nineveh to tell the people to repent. Jonah was in fear and did not think the Ninevites deserved forgiveness so he refused to go. He ended up being swallowed by a big fish. David, a man after God's own heart, committed adultery and murder! Everyone who committed sin in the Bible had to suffer the consequences, whether great or small. The same is true today. God wants obedience from His children.

"Do not be deceived, God is not mocked; for whatever a man sows, that he will also reap." (Galatians 6:7 NKJV)

Disobedience is such a great disappointment to God. It can ruin the very person God has called you to be. It also has the tendency to inflict emotional pain, bitterness, anger and unforgiveness on you and the people affected by your

Faith is not a

passion for

what is possible; rather,

a *requirement*

for the promised.

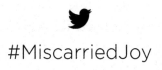

#MiscarriedJoy

decisions. Many pieces of our lives are determined by what we sow. Are you sowing good seeds or bad ones? The pleasures of the flesh are never worth the price you will be forced to pay for your disobedience. I wonder if Abraham and Sarah would have had to wait twenty-five years to have children had they walked in total obedience to God and submitted their lives and desires to have children to His plan. Our disobedience has the tendency to delay blessings in our lives. Disobedience can cause spiritual forces to block blessings in our lives. Satan works daily to deceive us into getting off of God's path and onto one that tickles the flesh, the one that feels good for a moment. But we will never reach our destiny and perfection in Christ through disobedience to His instruction. Does God still love you when you sin? Absolutely! God hates the sin but still extends His love through undeserving grace.

Have you ever assessed where you are spiritually and come to your own conclusion that you are walking in obedience to God's Word? If so, you become puzzled as to why you are still experiencing difficult challenges in those areas where you felt God should be blessing you? You may think, *"God, I am not killing, cheating, lying, fornicating, committing adultery or any other of those big sins that would definitely block blessings in my life."* I know I feel like this at times. I am committed to living my life for God. I have done what He has asked me to do. My husband and I kept ourselves until marriage. I study The Word, I spend time with God, I do what He instructs me to do. So it definitely seemed unfair to me that this is my journey to motherhood. I am often forced to remember that I must suffer for Christ, fair or unfair. Through many tribulations, we must enter the kingdom of God (Acts 14:22).

"For we wrestle not against flesh and blood, but against principalities, against powers, against the rulers of the darkness of this world, against spiritual wickedness in high places. Wherefore take unto you the whole armour of God, that ye may be able to withstand in the evil day, and having done all, to stand." (Ephesians 6:12-13 KJV)

If we are expecting God to come through for us, we must fulfill what He asks us to do. *"If you love me, you will keep my commandments"* (Luke 6:46 ESV). Can God trust you to fully glorify Him even in the middle of your storm? Please understand that your miscarriage, loss of your child or inability to conceive is not a result of your disobedience to God. Rather, obedience is a path we must continue to walk in because we love God and are submitted to His plan. As we make our requests known to Him, we should always go before Him with a pure heart and full intentions to be obedient to His Word and any direction He gives us for our lives. Our suffering is not random nor without purpose. Our greatest gifts are born out of our greatest pain. This suffering we are experiencing is our battleground. We can respond in two ways – one that curses God or one that continues to praise Him in the midst of what we are going through. The second option would be the one that obeys Him. Our obedience to Him will be far greater than our sacrifice for Him.

Trust God's Promises Over Your Own Ways

Can you imagine your natural father promising you something you've wanted forever and then it takes him twenty plus years to give it to you? Would you lose confidence

Neglecting to

trust God's *perfect* plan and

timing births Ishmaels - *seeds*

of the flesh - in our lives.

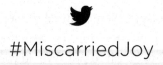

#MiscarriedJoy

in his promise or possibly trust him less, if at all? Wouldn't you grow frustrated waiting on your dad to do what he said? How many times would you ask, "Dad when are you going to fulfill your promise to me?" Wouldn't you remind him of what he said? I often wonder why Go allowed so much time to pass before fulfilling His promise to Abraham and Sarah. If God had done it expediently, maybe Sarah would not have gotten frustrated and allowed Hagar to sleep with her husband. How different would their lives have been if Sarah would have patiently waited for God to back up His word? You may, like me, have wondered how patient Sarah should have been. It did take twenty years for them to have the baby God had promised.

> *"But you must not forget this one thing, dear friends: A day is like a thousand years to the Lord, and a thousand years is like a day. The Lord isn't really being slow about his promise, as some people think. No, he is being patient for your sake. He does not want anyone to be destroyed, but wants everyone to repent." (2 Peter 3:8)*

Sarah wanted it to happen in her own timing. We can't criticize her for that because don't we do the same thing? Have you become frustrated with God's timing because it isn't according to your plan? Maybe you have been waiting for a baby for two years. Or maybe you have been in the waiting room for ten to fifteen years. God's way is not ours.

> *"My thoughts are nothing like your thoughts," says the Lord. 'And my ways are far beyond anything you could imagine. For just as the heavens are higher than*

the earth, so my ways are higher than your ways and my
thoughts higher than your thoughts." (Isaiah 55:8-9)

We act foolishly when we attempt to make His plans and purposes conform to ours. The proper course of action is to submit to His plan, His timing and His way.

I remember when I was single and wanted to be married very badly. I had a list of everything *I* wanted my husband to be. I wanted him to love God, be dark-skinned, about five feet ten inches or taller, have two degrees, a great corporate job, a great cook, handy around the house and know how to spiritually lead his family. I wanted to be the queen of his castle and work only because I wanted to and not because I had to. I wanted him to substantially provide all I needed and wanted. I prayed to be married so much that I thought God was probably tired of hearing me ask him to reveal my husband. I think I prayed for my husband for the very first time when I was about twenty-three. I didn't get married until I was thirty-three.

Most people would see this as ten years of waiting, but in reality it was ten years of God waiting on me. I dated men who I knew were not sent from God. I kept my very superficial list for a long time. I neglected to listen when God whispered, 'Tanika, he is not your husband,' and I ran back to a place of comfort out of fear of the unknown. I allowed the spirits of fear, doubt and impatience to operate in my life. In those ten years, God was waiting on me to surrender my own will and learn the lessons He was trying to teach me. I partly delayed my own blessing, but in the end, God's timing was so perfect. When I released what *I* wanted and was ready to accept His will for my life in this area, God showed up!

There is a season of preparation we must walk through for every blessing we receive in our lives. I was not ready to be a wife the first time I prayed for a husband. I had to learn to die to my selfish motives. I had to learn to stand firm when things get tough. God had to develop my prayer life, because who knew that I would end up praying for my husband more than I pray for myself? I had to become content being single if God never blessed me with a husband. Remember this, God will never bless us with something or someone we will prioritize above Him.

I wanted a husband so bad that had I been blessed with one in my twenties, I probably would not know God the way I do in my thirties. I know Him to be the lover of my soul; my lily in the valley; a way maker; my keeper; my provider; the One who rewards me; the God of mercy; the Most High God; the faithful God; the jealous God; the one and only true and living God; the God who never forgets about me, but hears me when I pray; the patient God; and the Father who wants to give me everything I desire according to His purpose for my life. I have seen God show up and show out in my life. So why would I think He wouldn't show up in this situation too? I suggest you reflect on how God has come through for you in the past. Has he spared your life? Was He the author of your love story? Has He healed you from anything? Hasn't He provided everything you need? Throw out all worry and doubt that God won't bless your life with the children you desire.

"That is why I tell you not to worry about everyday life — whether you have enough food and drink, or enough clothes to wear. Isn't life more than food, and your body more than clothing? Look at the birds. They don't plant or

harvest or store food in barns, for your heavenly Father feeds them. And aren't you far more valuable to him than they are? Can all your worries add a single moment to your life?

"And why worry about your clothing? Look at the lilies of the field and how they grow. They don't work or make their clothing, yet Solomon in all his glory was not dressed as beautifully as they are. And if God cares so wonderfully for wildflowers that are here today and thrown into the fire tomorrow, he will certainly care for you. Why do you have so little faith?" (Matthew 6:25-30)

God may not answer our prayers the way we want Him to, but He does answer them. So often, we are inclined to think that if God doesn't answer with a "yes," then He hasn't answered at all. What if His answer is "no" or "not right now?" God does not always give us what we want; He gives us what we need. Just as our parents did not fulfill every request we made, God does not respond to every prayer in the way we desire. It is still our responsibility to trust His plan over our own. It took Sarah thirteen years to finally surrender her will and learn the lessons God was trying to teach her. Sound familiar? She was walking in disbelief, a loss of faith, worry, fear and doubting God. But what I love that God never left her side. He was always there just as He is with us. Sarah was the one who attempted to fit her plans into God's plans. Despite her rebellion, God's promise never changed! Isn't that refreshing to know? When Abraham and Sarah surrendered their control and sat in the Presence of God, God delivered the news they would conceive (Genesis 18:10). A year later, they met their promised seed of the Spirit, Isaac.

What is it you have failed to surrender to God? We cannot put our hope and trust in our desire to have children, but in The God who creates life. God says, *"For I know the plans I have for you," says the LORD. "They are plans for good and not for disaster, to give you a future and a hope" (Jeremiah 29:11).* God's plans are so perfect and far better than anything we could imagine for ourselves. We don't know what our future holds; therefore, we must trust God to walk through every challenge with our heads held high, our hands in His and *"being confident of this, that he who began a good work in you will carry it on to completion until the day of Christ Jesus" (Philippians 1:6).* This temporary season of infertility or loss of a child is blessing you with an opportunity to know God in ways you have never known Him before. You will learn He wants the best for you. You will see that He keeps his promises. Just keep praying!

CHAPTER 4

In Due Time

"When Isaac was forty years old, he married Rebekah, the daughter of Bethuel the Aramean from Paddan-aram and the sister of Laban the Aramean.

Isaac pleaded with the LORD on behalf of his wife, *because she was unable to have children. The LORD answered Isaac's prayer, and Rebekah became pregnant with twins. But the two children struggled with each other in her womb. So she went to ask the LORD about it. "Why is this happening to me?" she asked.*

And the LORD told her, "The sons in your womb will become two nations. From the very beginning, the two nations will be rivals. One nation will be stronger than the other; and your older son will serve your younger son."

And when the time came to give birth, Rebekah discovered that she did indeed have twins!" (Genesis 25:20-24)

Everything happens in God's timing, according to His perfect plan. Isn't that just what you want to hear when you've been waiting and waiting for anything? Probably not. Living in a fast-paced society driven by immediate satisfaction, waiting is not something most of us enjoy. I mean who wants to wait for something you really want? Sitting in a line at the drive-thru waiting for your McDonald's order yields food. But is it the best food? Great quality requires a longer wait while special orders take more time.

My husband and I recently purchased our first home. Part of that process is decorating, purchasing furniture, landscaping and all those other things that come with home ownership. I have these grand ideas of how I want our house to look. My preference is to do everything all at once. However, it's not a wise financial decision, so we decided we would tackle one room at a time. It's driving me crazy because I want to do it all. Not now, but right now! But when I got married, I vowed to God that I would submit to my husband. Therefore, I must come under the leadership he has set for our home. It's the same when we receive the free gift of salvation.

We must submit to the authority, timing and ways of Jesus Christ. There will be things we don't agree with, assignments we don't want to accomplish, uninvited suffering we would rather not endure and times when we simply don't want to wait. But as His child, under His authority, we must relinquish control. A heart that is not submitted equates to a life that is unfilled. A heart that is willing to wait is a life that aligns perfectly with God's desires. How long are you willing to wait to get the very best God has for you?

Forty. If your twenty-year old self could visualize what life would be like at forty, what would you see? What would

A *heart* that is

not *submitted*

equates to a life

that is *unfilled*.

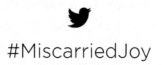

#MiscarriedJoy

you have accomplished? What are the plans you have (or had) for yourself? What interruptions have you encountered along the journey? Would it be your choice to wait until you turned forty to get married? What about giving birth to your first child at forty? I am willing to bet your answer to most, if not all, of these questions would be a solid *no*. There is a famous quote that says, *"If you want to make God laugh, tell him your plans."* I know with great certainty God has laughed at me. He laughed at me when I said I would get married by the age of twenty-seven and have all of my children by thirty. That clearly was not His plan for me. My love story went very differently from what I envisioned and well, you know about my journey to motherhood.

In Genesis, Chapter 24, we find one of the greatest love connections. As the story opens, Abraham's wife, Sarah, has died. Isaac has lost his mother and was probably in a state of grief and sorrow. Abraham knew his son would probably look for comfort in a woman (we are good at that!) and was concerned he may connect with a Canaanite woman. This would have a negative effect on the generations to come because the Canaanite people were idol worshippers. They practiced various manners of perversion similar to that found in Sodom and Gomorrah. As a father, Abraham felt responsible to help mold the generations to come and to protect his son from making a mistake that could have the wrong influence on future generations. So, he set the perfect love story in motion with God's guidance and dependence on His provision. He sent his servant to find a woman from his hometown, for He was certain they worshipped the One, True and Living God. The servant prayed and went to the well because he knew this was the place women came to draw water for their family. He sought the Lord's guidance and prayed that He would identify Isaac's wife by a sign.

> *"I will speak to a young woman. I'll say to her, 'Please lower your jar so I can have a drink.' Suppose she says, 'Have a drink of water, and I'll get some for your camels too.' Then let her be the one you have chosen for your servant Isaac. That's how I'll know you have been kind to my master." (Genesis 24:14)*

Rebekah showed great hospitality through her willingness to offer the servant a drink and enough for his camels as well. After meeting her family, the servant returned home with Rebekah. She and Isaac met in the field, their eyes met, they were immediately attracted to one another, and they went into the tent and married. God had prepared Rebekah's heart to receive Isaac. Their marriage was a holy set up for them to live happily ever after, except they didn't. The real love story in Genesis 24 is not just the one between Isaac and Rebekah, but the love of God toward His children and the immense regard for His promises.

THE STRUGGLE

Rebekah – a virgin, beautiful, courteous, resourceful, helpful, and hospitable. She had the qualities most men would dream of having in a wife. She went beyond what was expected and embodied the attitude of a servant (Genesis 24:15-25). Her initiative got her noticed. Her faith and courage motivated her to venture away from her comfort zone. She was the intended bride for Isaac and willingly left the familiar to travel to an unknown place to start a new life with her husband. She was a great source of comfort to Isaac after losing his mother, Sarah. The bible doesn't share much about their lives in the twenty-year span between their wedding day and the revelation of Rebekah being barren. But we can probably gather that they lived a life of unwavering faith, given they both had strong foundations in God before uniting as one. God rewarded her faithfulness with a monogamous marriage and removed her infertility as an answer to her husband's prayers.

"Isaac pleaded with the LORD on behalf of his wife, because she was unable to have children." (Genesis 25:21)

Isaac was a direct descendant of the man and woman blessed to be the father of many nations. His birth was the beginning of the manifestation of God's promise. The additional nations would be birthed through him. God said to Abraham, *"I will certainly bless you. I will multiply your descendants beyond number, like the stars in the sky and the sand on the seashore. Your descendants will conquer the cities of their enemies" (Genesis 22:17)*. If God made this promise, then certainly Isaac and Rebekah would not walk through the wilderness of infertility. Why would they, of all people, be temporarily unable to conceive? In Chapter 1, we learned that God is not the cause of our miscarriages or infertility, but he allows us to go through it. Just as the enemy taunted Job, he was out to do the same to Rebekah, to you and to me. The enemy is out to attack the seed. If he can pull up the root before it grows, he has less work to do on the earth. So he attempts to attack us through our seeds – the seeds of future generations, the seeds we sow into the ground and the seeds we sow into others. One seed brings about much fruit. If the enemy can attack the seed, his efforts will be effective for generations to come. Satan had foresight into the power and destiny of Abrahams's descendants. He knew they would lead into the lineage of Jesus Christ. It was his duty to put his greatest efforts towards preventing the perfect will of God from manifesting through Isaac and Rebekah. He was a high performer on his job then and he is still effective today.

But there is great news. He does not have the ability nor the power to defeat the children of God. *"I have given you authority to trample on snakes and scorpions and to overcome all the power of the enemy; nothing will harm you." (Luke 10:19)*. Though Satan can throw many obstacles our way, we have the authority to overcome everything. Our victory was already won through Jesus Christ and it manifests in our lives through prayer, faith and intimacy with God.

Isaac, the long-awaited answer to his parents' prayer for a child. He and Rebekah experienced the same fertility struggles as his parents, but handled the matter very differently. As we look back at his life, we can discern that he grew up knowing God and learning to trust Him. I believe he was fully aware of what was really occurring when Abraham took him up to Mount Moriah to offer him as a sacrifice to God (Genesis 22). He was gentle, a man of great patience and a man of prayer. He trusted that God was faithful to provide that which He had promised. When he found out Rebekah was having challenges conceiving, he never for a moment considered taking a concubine. Isaac went into prayer on behalf of his wife. He prayed and he waited on God to perform the miracle he was expecting. How long did it take? Twenty years to be exact. He was forty years old when

A heart that is

willing to wait is

a life that *aligns*

perfectly with

God's *desires*.

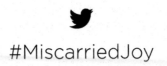

#MiscarriedJoy

he married his wife. "*...Isaac was sixty years old when Rebekah gave birth to them*" *(Genesis 25:26)*. Isaac and Rebekah prayed fervently and never stopped believing for their children! It took a lot of waiting and a lot of prayer. Isaac's patient faith was rewarded doubly – they gave birth to twin boys, Jacob and Esau. God was the matchmaker of this union, yet they still encountered trials which eventually made them stronger together and built a stronger bond between them and God. Isaac and Rebekah taught us that everything we desire according to God's will can be obtained through prayer.

"Just keep praying." This is often the response I receive when I share my story of Maurice and I wanting so badly to have children but are still waiting. I have prayed through the tears, the pain, the frustration, the great days and the not so good ones. I have prayed for God to open my womb. I know it is not His will to withhold any good thing from me (Psalm 84:11), but honestly, there are times when I don't know what else to pray. There are moments when doubt gets the very best of me and I neglect to pray for the children I desperately desire. I know how it feels to cry more than pray, to fear more than pray and even to have an array of hope greater than my diligence and sincerity to pray. The power of our prayers will only be as great as the level of our faith. We must believe the desires we bring to the feet of Jesus will manifest in our lives. Otherwise, why pray? I bet Rebekah felt the same way we do at times. Though Isaac was praying, Rebekah, being rooted in God, was undoubtedly praying too. She probably stayed on her face petitioning for children, even through those days when

she didn't have the motivation to confess her desires out of fear. I think that in her time with God, she carved out a special place to show gratitude to her praying husband. There is not much better in a relationship than a man that who covers you in prayer. Jacob and Esau were a reward for the prayers Isaac took to God in his secret place.

"Children are a gift from the Lord; they are a reward from him." (Psalm 127:3-5)

The secret place is where we learn the plans and purpose of God for our lives. Many times it is used as a "requesting room" where God's children bring their wants, desires and wishes to Him without any willingness to sacrifice anything. In my parents' home, many rewards came from my efforts of hard work. Honors grades resulted in extracurricular activities. Completing chores resulted in a weekly allowance. But there were many luxuries my parents gave us, not because of what we did, but because of their great love for us. There were times I received rewards I knew I did not deserve. I am so thankful that God *"has not dealt with us according to our sins, nor punished us according to our iniquities" (Psalm 102:10 NKJV)*. He is a Father who provides and gives us good gifts even when we don't deserve it. When I fail to give God the first fruit of my time, He still grants me with great rewards. When I fail to love others as God does, He still extends His grace. When I worry more than I pray, He still takes care of my needs. When my circumstances cause me to doubt, He is still trustworthy. When I don't treat God like the gracious and heavenly Father He is, He never ever leaves me nor forsakes me (Deuteronomy 31:6). We are beyond blessed to serve a God who doesn't *always* treat us according to what our motives and actions deserve. We must also remember that God gives us free will and if we continue to dishonor Him in any area of our lives, there will be consequences.

Isaac used his secret place and his private time to pray for his wife, Rebekah. Because he knew her heart, he felt her pain. She didn't have to repeatedly express her longing for a child. When you married your husband, the two of you joined as one flesh. When you pray for your spouse, you are also praying for yourself.

"For this reason a man will leave his father and mother and be united to his wife, and the two will become one flesh, so they are no longer two, but one flesh. Therefore, what God has joined together, let no one separate." (Matthew 19:5-6 NIV)

Isaac didn't just pray to the Lord. The scripture (Genesis 25:21) says he *pleaded* with The Lord. He made an emotional appeal, probably with a burdened heart and tear-filled eyes. Men are usually a bit more patient than women, except in the shopping mall. Given that Isaac *earnestly* prayed for God to grant their desire for children, we can deduce that Isaac too was tired of waiting. They were in their nineteenth year of marriage and still childless. I would have probably passed the checkpoint and thrown in the towel. But Isaac didn't. He laid out his heart before God on behalf of his wife. He prayed and kept waiting. Then, it finally happened in due time – in God's timing. The love story and the lives of Isaac and Rebekah encompass some very powerful lessons of faith. They waited with great patience, not because they wanted a baby, but because they welcomed God to develop the Fruits of the Spirit in their lives.

The *power* of our

prayers will only be

as *great* as the

level of our *faith*.

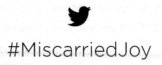

#MiscarriedJoy

A Praying Husband is a Powerful Husband

In the book, *The Power of a Praying Husband*, Stormie Omartian makes a powerful comparison that sticks out in my mind. She compared wives to automobiles. Here is an excerpt of what she says:

> Your wife is like an automobile. She may be high maintenance like an Italian sports car. She might be as refined and expensive as a German luxury sedan. She may be solid and sturdy like an SUV, or delicate like a Pebble Beach Concours d'Elegance show car. She could be an efficient six-cylinder type, or be a faster but costlier V-8 model. She may be dependable in all kinds of weather like a four-wheel drive, or she may have no downhill traction control at all, even on a good day. Whatever she is, whether she is tiny like a compact car or full-size and beyond, she needs fuel to make her run smoothly.[5]

What a powerful comparison! I am known for running so fast and quickly becoming overwhelmed, attempting to run on my own fuel rather than the fuel of the Holy Spirit. I never anticipated that life as a woman and a wife would require so much of me. I thought getting married was going to make life easier. In many ways it did, but in other ways, it required more than I imagined. I learned that I had to pray and study God's Word more, develop a deeper intimacy with The Father and be spiritually armed to fight against the enemy. The moment we said "I do" was the moment Satan strategized his attacks on our lives. He attacked our marriage in many ways.

God built women to be nurturing, to put others before ourselves, to juggle many tasks, and sometimes we feel we can do it all. So we start with full tanks, attempt to do it all, run until the fuel is gone and fumes are the only thing keeping us moving. Does this sound familiar to you? or am I the only in the world like this? I often find that when I am overwhelmed with life, I am undernourished with the strength of God. Remember I talked about that secret place? Well that is also the perfect location to receive the strength of God. When we neglect to get into His Presence, we slowly deplete our fuel and run on empty. Stormie Omartian also says, *If a woman doesn't spend enough time every day with the Lord in prayer, worship and the Word of God, she will lose ground and the enemy of her soul will run her down.*[6]

Run down has been the perfect description for my emotions during many moments in this journey. Not a day goes by when I don't think about our angel babies, imagine our next pregnancy, think about baby names or anxiously await the twenty-ninth day of my cycle to take a pregnancy test. Yes, it can be consuming at times. Those are the moments when I not only need God, but I also need my husband to remind me to just enjoy the journey of life while waiting in peace. You see, I have been labeled a control freak, but this journey has reminded me that God has control over all things. I cannot create life nor can I rush the process. I am so grateful for my husband in these times because he covers me in prayer when I don't have the wherewithal to pray for myself. He is the first to see the tears well up in my eyes when a woman shares her recent miscarriage or struggle to conceive.

My heart aches in a similar way as the day we discovered that our babies' souls had gone to heaven, and he immediately feels my pain. A man has a very special role and a huge responsibility in marriage and also in this season we are facing. You are not meant to go through this alone, neither emotionally nor spiritually. Your husband should be on the front line of this spiritual war between you and the enemy. Most of the biblical stories of barren women place more emphasis on the woman, but not with Isaac and Rebekah. There isn't one verse in the bible where we see Rebekah communicating with God regarding her desire to be a mother. I think God divinely placed this example in His Word so we could visualize the power of our husbands' prayers and the significance of his role as the head of our homes. God responds to the prayers of our husbands, especially when we don't have the strength to utter our needs to God.

"But there is one thing I want you to know: The head of every man is Christ, the head of woman is man, and the head of Christ is God." (1 Corinthians 11:3)

"Husbands, love your wives, just as Christ loved the church and gave himself up for her to make her holy, cleansing her by the washing with water through the word..." (Ephesians 5:22-23 NIV)

God made husbands the head of the home and has given them authority over all power of the enemy (Luke 19:10). God placed ultimate responsibility with respect to the marriage and household on the shoulders of the husband. They are in a position of leadership and should use their authority especially when the enemy sets out to attack their wives and families. Prayer is a direct connection to heaven. When our husbands pray for us we are immediately put in a posture to receive. Infertility has a tendency to negatively affect marriages, relationships and friendships. The tensions become stressful, the emotions become taxing and the pain becomes easier to take out on someone else rather than dealing with it. Our husbands, parents, siblings and friends wish there was something they could do to take the pain away, but there isn't. Only God can heal you from the inside out. But they can ease our burdens through their prayers on our behalf.

I lived on my own for almost fifteen years before getting married. Needless to say, allowing my husband to totally lead was quite the adjustment for me. I was used to carrying every load on my own. I rarely asked for help and if I was going through any type of emotional struggle, I often kept it between me and God. When I got married, I had to learn to share the most intimate pieces of me with someone else. It did not happen overnight. My best friend will tell you that I am like a vault. It is so hard to get the code from me to open secret details of my life. In fact, many people knew I am writing a book, but only a handful of people even knew what it is about. I am just that private.

But what I've learned through marriage is that keeping it all in does two things that are detrimental to our physical and emotional health – it greatly increases our level of stress and decreases the power of our prayers. *"For where two or three gather together as my followers I am there among them."* *(Matthew 18:20).* As wives, we are not meant to carry any burden alone. I often kept my emotions to myself after our

When I am

overwhelmed

with life, I am

undernourished

with the strength

of God.

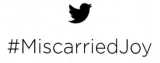

#MiscarriedJoy

first miscarriage because I didn't want to bother my husband or make him sad just because I was having a bad day. But he knew what I was feeling, he could hear the tears over the phone and my pain was his pain. He was hurting because I was hurting.

My pain brought him to his knees in prayer. Now we pray together daily for our children. He prays to God that my womb will be opened to bear the promised fruit of the generations coming behind us. He prays that the memories of my pain would be used for purpose and the hurt would be erased. He prays that the seeds we sow into others will sprout up in our lives. He prays when I have nothing left to say. When I have nothing left to give, no encouragement to pass on and no words to describe my frustration, he prays. When I wonder if it will ever happen or have moments when I want to think about the "what ifs," he prays. The sound of his prayers over me calms my soul and relieves my anxiety. The tears that fill my eyes are diminished when he prays for me. There is just something about the sheer embrace and voice of my husband's prayers that is unexplainable. The Bible instructs us to *"Give all your worries and cares to God, for He cares for you."*

Carrying the stress, worry and anxiety is a clear indication that we do not trust God with every detail of our lives. I asked God why I would feel such tranquility when I released my feelings to my husband and held his hand in prayer. He revealed that when I release my stress to my husband, I am showing him I trust him with my life. It takes an ultimate level of humility as a former "independent woman" to recognize my husband wants to meet my needs and is willing to carry my burdens. I quickly learned that every worry I bring to Maurice, he takes to God in prayer. He is essentially the conduit of easing my burdens to God when I don't have the energy to carry them to His feet. This is what Isaac did for Rebekah, and it is what our husbands should be doing for us. If you, like me, don't want to place a load on your husband with your emotions regarding having children one day, give it to Jesus. God made our husbands stronger than us to carry weight we aren't strong enough to sustain.

> *"In the same way, you husbands must give honor to your wives. Treat your wife with understanding as you live together. She may be weaker than you are, but she is your equal partner in God's gift of new life. Treat her as you should so your prayers will not be hindered." (1 Peter 3:7)*

Just as your husband would be coaching and praying for you during labor, he should be doing the same in the spirit as you wait on God to conceive and birth the children you are believing Him for. There is something so powerful in a praying husband, especially when he goes to God on your behalf. Our husbands see every emotion we feel throughout this journey. They are there to wipe the tears, speak life, encourage us, and are often the voice reminding us that God is faithful!

EMBRACE PEACE IN HIS TIMING

Abraham and Sarah waited twenty-five years before Isaac was born. Isaac and Rebekah waited twenty years before the birth of Jacob and Esau. God was faithful in what He promised, and it came in due time. I would venture to say both couples exercised great patience. Let's have an honest moment here. Am I the only one that hates the statement:

"All in God's timing." I mean what about that is comforting? When someone says this, they are essentially telling me to "just keep waiting." Okay, let me get this straight. First I have to keep praying and then I have to keep waiting? "Jesus, how long do I have to wait?" I am tired of waiting. I am exhausted with the monthly pregnancy tests that are negative. I don't want to think about when or if I am ovulating. I want babies! It is completely fine to vent to God. But even in the midst of the time pressures we place on ourselves, God is not moved by our emotions. He is moved by our faith!

> *"Be still in the presence of the Lord, and wait patiently for him to act." (Psalm 37:7)*

In pursuing your dreams, callings and even the purpose of God, we will be faced with delays. I think we all have been in waiting rooms countless times. A few weeks ago I went to the doctor for my annual visit. I arrived about twenty minutes early for my four o'clock appointment. I knew it would take me at least fifteen minutes to complete the necessary new patient paperwork. I turned in the forms with about five minutes to spare before my set appointment time. I found myself waiting much longer than I anticipated and far longer than what I felt was professional. I approached the check-in desk to inquire why I was waiting for so long. Her response was "the doctor is still with another patient." I became a bit agitated and, for a moment, considered rescheduling because I had something to do. This waiting was eating into my scheduled plans and I didn't have any time for delays or interruptions.

Against the judgment of my flesh, I continued to wait peacefully. I knew this appointment was a crucial one in our journey to becoming parents and since it was important, I could either welcome the delay with a positive attitude or put it off until later and possibly be forced to wait again in the future. The office closed at five o'clock, so I was cognizant of a timeframe. I was certain within the next hour, my appointment will have concluded and I would be on my way to the next mission of my day.

But the spiritual waiting room is much different because we tend to make appointments during a window of time that is convenient for us, often receiving little consultation from God. So we arrive in the spiritual waiting room expecting no delay at all. We want to be called into the exam room at the exact time we, not God, made the appointment. The lives we have envisioned in our minds are the lives *we* want to manifest on earth. Rarely do we warmly welcome delays with positive attitudes, pure motives and genuine requests for God to prepare us to walk in peace in this season. We murmur, complain, we cry more than we pray, we fall into comparison and we doubt. "God, did you forget about me, your favorite, your beloved child in whom you are well pleased?"

Jesus uses these delays to prepare, test and develop us to successfully face and overcome obstacles in the next phase of building our faith. He knows our faith will be tested in larger manners than our current circumstances. He knows we will need more strength to endure what is coming in our future. This season of waiting, my dear sister, is a season for us to learn and experience the divine character of God in ways we would have never known if it weren't for *this*. God is teaching us that we must not only wait, but we must wait in peace.

"Enthusiasm without knowledge is not good; impatience will get you into trouble." (Proverbs 19:2 GNT)

Isn't it frustrating when our timing doesn't align with God's timing? I am thirty-five years old and am told by doctors that I am now in the high-risk zone to have children. This scientific fact could cause me to be in a great hurry to conceive. Honestly, it was once a root cause in my rush to have children. I once wondered if my age meant anything to God. Silly me! How old was Sarah? Ninety! But I don't want to be Sarah or Rebekah. I want to be a mother before I am forty. Don't you want the same? Well, here's the reality. God was not moved by Isaac and Rebekah's age and He is not moved by our age, scientific facts or pregnancy risks. *"But you must not forget this one thing, dear friends: A day is like a thousand years to the Lord, and a thousand years is like a day. The Lord isn't really being slow about his promise, as some people think" (2 Peter 3:8-9a).* God is so much larger than time and we can't make Him move faster than He plans. We must rest and wait patiently and peacefully for Him to act. *"You saw me before I was born. Every day of my life was recorded in your book. Every moment was laid out before a single day had passed" (Psalm 139:16).*

*"But the Holy Spirit produces this kind of fruit in our lives: love, joy, **peace**, **patience**, kindness, goodness, faithfulness, gentleness, and self-control." (Galatians 5:22)*

The Holy Spirit is our helper and our faith in God is the best strategy to successfully endure and overcome this temporary inability to successfully conceive, carry and birth children. The fruits of the Spirit are developed in us through the continual and spontaneous work of The Holy Spirit *in* us. These fruits are the very nature of Jesus Christ. As we continue this walk, we should become more like Him. These characteristics are obtained through building intimacy with the Holy Spirit. It happens when we join our lives, our timing and our desires to Jesus. This means embracing peace and resting in His plan.

"And the peace of God, which transcends all understanding, will guard your hearts and your minds in Christ Jesus." (Philippians 4:7 NIV)

True peace is not found in our ability to remain positive or in control of our feelings. It comes from knowing God is in control. It is what guards our hearts against any anxiety. Merriam-Webster Dictionary defines peace as *"a state of tranquility or quietness; freedom from disquieting, oppressive thoughts or emotions; harmony."*[7] Holy Scripture describes peace as a gift from God and being harmonious to His character. To know God is to live in His peace, which is not circumstantial. It is everlasting and we can live in it regardless of what is occurring around us. This world is in total chaos, but because we serve God, we can live in peace in the midst. Because we are kingdom citizens, we receive all of the gifts and benefits from our Father. Our character is not only developed in the waiting but also in *how* we wait.

"Who may ascend the mountain of the Lord? Who may stand in his holy place? The one who has **clean hands and a pure heart,** *who does not trust in an idol or swear by a false god. They will receive blessing from the Lord and vindication from God their Savior." (Psalm 24:3-5)*

"May God himself, the God of peace, sanctify you through and through. May your whole spirit, soul and body be kept blameless at the coming of our Lord Jesus Christ. The one who calls you is faithful, and he will do it." (1 Thessalonians 5:23-24)

The fruits of the *Spirit*

are developed in us

through the *continual*

and spontaneous work of the

Holy Spirit in us.

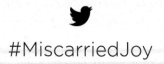

#MiscarriedJoy

This time of development is meant to develop the fruits of patience and peace, but also to take an inward look at our lives. This challenge is a key ingredient to our sanctification. Why? Because as we go through it, we are developing the fruits of The Spirit. We are exchanging fear for faith, anxiety for peace, frustration for patience and jealousy for joy. How can we become more like Christ? By eliminating those inner traits that do not align with His character. The gifts God gives to us are often left on the table due to our refusal to submit. We know His will by knowing His Word and seeking His wisdom in all things. Recognize that developing these fruits are a process. When you plant a corn seed, you don't wake up and see full ears of corn. It is a process.

"First the stalk, then the head, then the full kernel in the head." (Mark 4:28)

A process requires multiple steps and it is rare that great changes happen quickly. Ladies, we must go through the waiting process. Embrace longsuffering with an attitude of peace and blessings will be the reward. Don't run from this experience. Let patience have its perfect work in you. Isaac and Rebekah peacefully remained in the waiting season. God blessed them doubly!

FIND REST ALONG THE JOURNEY

As we develop patience, God promises us we will be complete, lacking nothing (James 1:4). *"Suffering produces perseverance; perseverance character; and character, hope" (Romans 5:4 NIV)*. We learn to trust God through experiences that require a deeper level of faith each time. When I first met my best friend, Mary, we were just coworkers. Both of us being from Michigan ignited a common spark that instantly connected us. The first time she came to my house, we both had our guards up because we didn't *know* each other. As we spent more time together, we began to know one another intimately. As we endured hardships in our lives separately or together, we gained a great level of trust each time. Today, I trust her with the deepest secrets of my heart. In fact, I trust her with my life. But this did not happen overnight. It took seasons of overcoming obstacles together. It is the same way with building our trust in Jesus Christ. Challenges in our lives to give us opportunities to build our patience, faith, trust and hope in Him. We see His faithfulness through our patience. Each time He delivers, we let go of trusting ourselves and trust Him.

If God did everything we asked for instantaneously, we would never grow and develop in our spirituality. God gives us desires, hopes and dreams, but He doesn't always give us knowledge of the exact timing of His plan. We might give up if we knew how long it would take. But we stay in the game because there is a chance it could happen at any moment. Peace comes only through trusting God. I won't lose sleep wondering when we will conceive again. I won't fear if my next pregnancy will be viable. I will place every single burden, fear and question at the feet of Jesus. He is a good Father and I know He desires to bless me with all good things as I walk according to His will. There are days when I wish Rebekah was my friend so she can encourage me in the wait. But I have a greater friend in Jesus that keeps me strong through the pressure.

Would you still trust God's timing if you were in your nineteenth year of waiting for a child? Would you bask in the peace of God knowing that He who promised is faithful? Would you give up and do things your own way? Isaac and Rebekah must have surely considered it. You see, in those times, fertility treatments and adoption were not options for barren women. That had one choice: pray and rest. That is exactly what they did. Isaac *pleaded* with God. They never succumbed to the pressure to give up.

If you have ever been hiking, you know you must take moments to rest during the excursion. During those breaks, you often look back to see how far you have come. You look down to see how far you have climbed. Though the journey may be challenging, it is peaceful. The sounds of the birds chirping, the bright sun shining down leaving just enough shade to keep you cool, and maybe the flow of the ocean river all brings a calm during your climb. You won't get tired or lose stamina as long as you find rest along the way. You may not know exactly how long it will take to get to the top, but because you have climbed so far, you may as well keep going. Once you get to the top, you can rest because the journey back down is much easier. You know the route, the obstacles, where to hold on and where to let go. You know you will make it, because God has kept you covered along the way. So, you take your time, you trust the journey and you rest. It is the same way in our trials.

Whether you are waiting for children, a new job, financial increase in your family or even healing in your marriage, nothing will get better until you decide to give it all over to Jesus and rest. God never sleeps nor slumbers so why should you lose sleep or neglect your rest when the Master who controls all has it in His hands?

I look up to the mountains – does
my help come from there?
² My help comes from the LORD,
who made heaven and earth!

³ He will not let you stumble;
the one who watches over you will not slumber.
⁴ Indeed, he who watches over Israel
never slumbers or sleeps.

⁵ The LORD *himself watches over you!*
The LORD *stands beside you as your protective shade.*
⁶ The sun will not harm you by day,
nor the moon at night.

⁷ The LORD *keeps you from all harm*
and watches over your life.
⁸ The LORD *keeps watch over you as you come*
and go, both now and forever. (Psalm 121)

Resting is an act of faith. It signals to God that you are waiting *in faith*. I am reminded of the time Jesus and His disciples were on a boat. A big storm made its way to the boat. The disciples were trembling with fear. The ship was being tossed, waves were breaking into the boat and it began to fill with water. Where was Jesus when all of this was happening? He was asleep! The first time I read this story, I was astounded that Jesus could sleep through a storm like this. I imagine they weren't traveling on *Royal Caribbean Harmony of the Seas*. They must have felt every wave and some may have experienced motion sickness. Jesus, their protector, was sleeping!

"Jesus was sleeping at the back of the boat with his head on a cushion. The disciples woke him up, shouting, "Teacher, don't you care that we're going to drown?" When Jesus woke up, he rebuked the wind and said to the waves, "Silence! Be still!" Suddenly the wind stopped, and there was a great calm. Then he asked them, "Why are you afraid? Do you still have no faith?" (Mark 4:38-40)

I jump up when I hear thunder or the torrential pouring of rain, so sleeping through a storm on what may have been a sail boat? That definitely would not have been me. Jesus was able to rest comfortably in the midst of an intense storm because He had the peace of God. He was fully confident God would rescue Him and protect Him even in the middle of the storm. Others may be harmed, but not Jesus and His disciples. Even the winds obey God! When we get into a storm, we have the human tendency to fret, lose sleep and worry if we will ever experience life on the other side of it. This is an obvious sign that you are not living by faith.

If you are lacking peace and joy, you are not trusting God. If you are focusing on *when* while not enjoying *now*, you are not trusting God. "Jesus where is the rainbow after this storm?" It is coming, my friend. You must rest. There are so many medical pressures the doctors can place on us, whether it be age or other medical conditions that stand in the way of us having babies. When Jesus was crucified, so were all of those sicknesses and challenges that prevent us from doing what God created our bodies to do. It is our job to pray and peacefully rest in His promises.

When Rebekah left her family to become Isaac's wife, her family blessed her with these words: *"May you, our sister, become the mother of many thousands of children."* I can imagine the smile on her face when she heard those words. She probably couldn't wait to call home with the news that they were expecting. It is probably the same feeling I had when my family would tell me how much they were looking forward to us having children. There is little I want more than to bless my husband with children, tell my parents they will officially be Gran Gran and Papa, and bring excitement to my sisters with the news they will be aunties. I had such an exciting way to tell family about the twins I was carrying, but I never got the chance to do so. When the second pregnancy happened, I was ecstatic to share the news, but I didn't get to share a good report. Rebekah had to wait two decades before she could inform her family she was expecting. Even in that, she rested. We, too, must rest in the promises of God.

CHAPTER 5

Birthing Contentment

What if? Is that a question you've asked yourself at some point in your journey of waiting? I surely have. Not with an attitude of doubt, but rather with a heart towards contentment. *What if?* What if your life remained the same as it is today? What if some of your deepest desires remained unfulfilled? What if your marriage remained the same? What if God has you where He wants you to be, but keeps you there longer than you've ever wanted to stay? Would you still serve God? Would you still trust Him? Would you still give Him your unending devotion? What if? Honestly, I have asked myself the question none of us want to be faced with, "What if I never give birth to children?" The Holy Spirit brought this question to me in my quiet place. I believe it was more of a heart check, rather than what my or your reality will be. God wants to know we are serving Him out of genuineness and not selfish motives to get what we want. In the book of Philippians, Paul said *"for I have learned to be content whatever the circumstances. I know what it is to be in need, and I know what it is to have plenty. I have learned the secret of being content in any and every situation, whether well fed or hungry, whether living in plenty or in want" (Philippians 4:11-12).*

If God never fulfills your desire to birth children, what will you do? How will you react? Will you allow bitterness and discontentment to take root in your heart? Will you become jealous of every pregnant friend or family member? Will you envy every mother you come across? Paul learned to be content whether he had plenty or whether he was in need. This is only accomplished by relying on Jesus' power for strength.

I love the story of the thorn in Paul's flesh sent by a messenger of Satan to torment him. He never made it clear what the thorn was, but only told us it was there. It could have been a sickness, disease or a spiritual battle he was forced to fight daily. Whatever it was, I know it was debilitating, bothersome and painful. Can you imagine a thorn from a rose stuck in any part of your flesh and you are unable to remove it? Ouch! I imagine Paul's thorn was much worse than that. Paul said *"Three times I pleaded with the Lord to take it away from me. But he said to me, 'My grace is sufficient for you, for my power is made perfect in weakness.' Therefore, I will boast all the more gladly about my weaknesses, so that Christ's power may rest on me. That is why, for Christ's sake, I delight in weaknesses, in insults, in hardships, in persecutions, in difficulties. For when I am weak, then I am strong" (2 Corinthians 12:9).*

Paul prayed three times for God to remove it, but He left it there. How many times have you prayed for God to open your womb or keep your baby healthy to term? But still, God has not done it *yet*. I am sure this thorn was a hindrance to Paul's assignment, but he still fulfilled it. Why? Because though he did not receive manifestation of his healing, the gifts bestowed upon him were so much greater than the thorn in his side. He received an immense amount of God's grace, development of his character, an increased sense of humility and the ability to empathize with others.

Those are the characteristics needed to walk out God's calling in your life. I can inspire and encourage other women experiencing challenges with conceiving and having children because it has been the thorn in my side. It has made me stronger spiritually, has taught me great patience and has given me the opportunity to feel what women like you are feeling. I can cry with you, share sentimental moments, exchange memories of walking into the operating room and unite with you in prayer. I can effectively sympathize with you, and so can Rachel.

Every woman has a friend she calls for specific purposes. We have that friend who makes us laugh, the one that is always ready to fight on your behalf, the one who keeps us in order, the one that will cry with you, the one that will tell you what you want to hear, and the one you never want to call when your husband is wrong and you are right because she is going to give you the hard truth.

Rachel would be the unhappy, envious friend; the one who is always complaining, comparing and competing. When we first meet her in Genesis 29, she is tending her father's sheep. Jacob noticed her from a short distance and immediately became attracted to her beauty. Because he was Laban's nephew, he was welcomed into their home where he stayed for a whole month. He got to see Rachel day in and day out. After a month, he was surely in love with her. How do I know? Because he offered to work for Laban for seven

Envy is initiated at

the exact place where

discontentment

is interrupted.

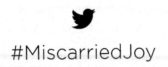

#MiscarriedJoy

years in exchange for Rachel's hand in marriage. That is a long time to chase a woman! So he worked for seven years, though it *"seemed like only a few days because of his love for her"* *(Genesis 29:20)*. But there is a twist. Laban deceived Jacob and gave Leah to him in the evening because she was the oldest. Jacob was unaware of the custom of the land that the older daughter be married first. He was furious! Laban agreed to give him Rachel too, in exchange for another seven years of work. Fourteen years and one week of work is what Jacob gave to get the love of his life.

> *"Laban replied, "It is not our custom here to give the younger daughter in marriage before the older one. Finish this daughter's bridal week; then we will give you the younger one also, in return for another seven years of work."*
>
> *And Jacob did so. He finished the week with Leah, and then Laban gave him his daughter Rachel to be his wife. Laban gave his servant Bilhah to his daughter Rachel as her attendant. Jacob made love to Rachel also, and his love for Rachel was greater than his love for Leah. And he worked for Laban another seven years." (Genesis 29:26-30 NIV)*
>
> *Jacob had two wives, but he loved Rachel more! "When the Lord saw that Leah was not loved, he opened her womb but Rachel was barren." (Genesis 29:31 NIV)*

Growing up with sisters has to be one of the best experiences of my life. I was the only child for twelve years and I did not enjoy it too much. I never had anyone at home to play with, so it may not be a surprise to you that I had a few imaginary friends in my time. My mom had some issues conceiving after I was born. In fact, doctors told her that she would never be able to have children again. I prayed often for God to bless me with siblings. I actually wanted a brother so I could be my daddy's only girl, but instead God gave me twin sisters. Do you see how He crushed that spirit of selfishness in me at an early age? On September 29, 1993, my life changed forever. There were two five pound babies who instantly filled my life with immense joy. Everything about them was, and still is, beautiful. Holding them in my arms was physical evidence that what we war for spiritually can happen in the natural.

As sisters, we share everything. Our genetic makeups are similar, elements of our personalities are related and most people can look at us and tell that we are definitely sisters. We share secrets we will take to our graves. There isn't much I wouldn't do for those ladies. In the midst of each pregnancy loss, it was those, *"Nika, you are going to be okay;" "Nika, I love you;" and "Nika, I am praying for you"* calls that helped me to be stronger than I ever thought I could be. Their encouragement was a healing balm to my heart. I love this quote from Mary Montagu: *"There can be no situation in life in which the conversation of my dear sister will not administer some comfort to me."* A sister's love is a blessing from God!

Leah and Rachel were sisters. They probably shared everything my sisters and I have shared over the years. I am sure they laughed, cried and got into big trouble together. Isn't that what sisters do? Oh yeah, they had many sibling rivalries in their lifetime, too. Rachel, being the younger sister, probably looked up to Leah. Maybe she wanted to wear her clothes, stole her makeup, read her diary and those other behaviors of younger siblings. But when it was time

Seasons of *waiting*

reveal our true

motives and builds

our *commitment*

to God's plan.

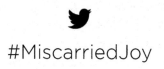

#MiscarriedJoy

to get married, Rachel was noticed first, but Leah took her man! I believe this is what planted the seed of jealousy in their relationship. They were married to the same man, which ignited the spirit of competition in Rachel, especially when she realized that Leah was super fertile and she was not able to conceive.

Can you imagine what it's like to watch your sister having baby after baby by the man who loves you more? I can't! I would be furious. I would be hurt. I too would be jealous of my own sister. My flesh just may win that battle, and then I would have to repent. Living in constant comparison to her beautiful sister Rachel, Leah was not hidden from God's love and concern. God opened the flood gates of her womb. Leah had given birth to Reuben, Simeon, Levi and Judah. Rachel had four nephews but still no children. Leah's position as Jacob's wife had been affirmed through her ability to give him children. Rachel felt useless. Her suffering worsened as time passed and with each moment she witnessed Leah enjoying life with her sons.

"When Rachel saw that she was not bearing Jacob any children, she became jealous of her sister. So she said to Jacob, "Give me children, or I'll die!" Jacob became angry with her and said, "Am I in the place of God, who has kept you from having children?" Then she said, "Here is Bilhah, my servant. Sleep with her so that she can bear children for me and I too can build a family through her." So she gave him her servant Bilhah as a wife. Jacob slept with her, and she became pregnant and bore him a son." (Genesis 30:1-5 NIV)

Rachel's heart-felt words to Jacob were overflowing with desperation and agony. She simply wanted to fulfill her destiny as a wife and a mother, but God had not opened her womb. Rachel, similar to Sarah, attempted to "help God out" by giving Bilhah to Jacob to bear children for her. Bilhah produced two children for Rachel. She now felt vindicated and satisfied. Her attempts to outdo her sister pushed Leah over the edge and started one of greatest sibling rivalries in the Bible. After Leah had given birth to her four boys, her womb was closed. But because she wanted to compete with her sister to win Jacob's love, she gave her servant, Zilpah, to Jacob. She gifted him with two additional sons.

The sisters were in a cruel competition and in their race to see who could have the most children (as if this were a sign of Jacob's love for them), they both gave Jacob a concubine. Though Bilhah had given Jacob children, Rachel must have still felt a room of emptiness in her heart. She still had not been blessed with the opportunity to birth Jacob's child herself. Oh what an incredible pain. I know that she, like us, must have cried every twenty-eight days upon the discovery that she still had not conceived.

She hurled her anger towards Jacob. *"Give me children, or I'll die!"* she cried. But she was asking something of Jacob that only God could perform. Her season of waiting was atrocious. Instead of becoming better, she became bitter. Instead of basking in joy, she tottered in jealousy. She even failed to realize that her husband's devotion to her was interdependent of her ability to have children. Her envy and competitive spirit tarnished the loving relationship she once had with her sister. Rachel was discontent, which led her to make mistakes we should learn from and be careful not to repeat in our lives.

Eliminating Envy

*"For wherever there is jealousy and selfish
ambition, there you will find disorder
and evil of every kind. (James 3:16)*

In today's world, wealth, business or professional success
fulfill the requirements for happiness. When people don't
feel accomplished in various areas of their lives, jealousy
arises and they become sad or even angry at what others
have achieved. Jealousy destroys relationships as it did with
Rachel and Leah. For some reason, whenever I am in a
waiting season, it seems like God puts me in position to be
around those who are experiencing the exact thing for which
I am praying. When I was believing God for my husband,
I got wind of every proposal (well, it seems like it) and I
was invited to wedding after wedding. Now that my husband
and I are praying for children, baby news is delivered to
me day after day in my circle of friends and definitely all
down my social media feed. There are so many immediate
opportunities for me to become jealous.

God is presenting me with a choice. I could choose to
envy the joy of others or I can choose to rejoice for what God
is doing in their lives. The more we focus on ourselves and
our own desires, the less we focus on God. Jealousy prevents
us from comprehending that *all* gifts are apportioned by
The Father according to His wisdom. We should choose to
genuinely celebrate others, void of any selfish ambition. Not
too many women would openly admit they are jealous but,
secretly, there probably have been times when each of us
has envied some element of someone else's life. Rachel was
jealous of her own sister! She was initially content knowing

that Jacob loved her more. But all hell broke loose when Leah proved to be the wife that could fulfill every man's dream – having not just one son, but four! Envy is initiated at the exact place where discontentment is interrupted.

"For I envied the arrogant when I saw the prosperity of the wicked." (Psalm 73:3 NIV)

The psalmist in the scripture above became envious when he took his eyes off of what God has purposed and set apart for him and began to want what others have. Coveting has become a strong part of our culture. Everyone obtains more and then wants more. It is a vicious cycle that forces people to value things more than the God that created *all things*. Jealousy, a work of the flesh, is often the result of pride and self-centeredness. It prevents you from becoming an advocate for a friend and instead leads you towards becoming a rival. God's perfect love is one that encourages, uplifts and celebrates His blessings. Some think the waiting season is a direct result of what we have done or may have failed to do. This is sometimes false. God does not have you waiting because you have not prayed enough. Your waiting may not even be connected to your obedience. He definitely doesn't have you waiting because He forgot about you. God has us waiting because He wants to develop something in each of us. Seasons of waiting reveals our true motives and builds our commitment to God's plan. If jealousy is in our heart, it will emerge in the wait. If discontentment is buried in your spirit, it will surface in your wait. God is building your character while you are waiting. This wait is for a divine purpose. The longer we focus on someone else's blessings, the longer we will wait for our own.

Jealously is a *thief*.

It steals the

opportunity to

celebrate the greatest

gifts from God

with the *people* we love.

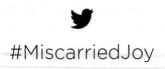

\#MiscarriedJoy

I have been told, *"Tanika, you have the perfect life,"* to which I often laugh. If only they knew! It may seem that way to some looking from the outside, but once you get past the fog-stained windows, you will see my life is not perfect in any way. I have felt alone. I have struggled with knowing my purpose. I have had struggles in my marriage. There is nothing easy about mending two very different historical creations. There have been moments where we felt more like oil and water. In addition to that, two miscarriages in less than a year does not seem like a life someone would choose. Month after month of negative pregnancy tests when you *know* a child will be conceived in love, is everything but a joyful experience. When you take off the rose-colored glasses, you will see everything *except* a perfect life.

I am willing to bet no woman would choose this waiting season on her own. There is no such thing as a perfect life. And guess what? The woman whom you think has the perfect life because she had the babies you yearn for, well, her life isn't perfect either. Maybe she too had multiple miscarriages. Maybe she had to give birth to a baby that didn't survive. Maybe she is in debt because of the large investment her and her husband chose to make for In-Vitro Fertilization. Maybe the babies she totes around had to be birthed by someone else. Maybe she is having marital issues because the babies are taking a toll on the marriage that wasn't strong enough to handle an additional load. You may want her outcome, but you surely don't want every piece of her journey. This is why we cannot envy what we see from the outside. Your journey is yours and hers belongs to her.

God knew we would fall into comparison. I believe that is why He gave us the tenth commandment *"You must not covet your neighbor's house. You must not covet your neighbor's wife, male or female servant, ox or donkey, or anything else that belongs to your neighbor" (Exodus 20:17).* Jealousy and envy result in bitterness, discontentment and a lack of thankfulness.

When we allow roots of bitterness to grow in our lives, we slowly destroy the inner peace God has provided. *"See to it that no one falls short of the grace of God and that no bitter root grows up to cause trouble and defile many" (Hebrews 12:15).* Bitterness corrupts all those involved, starting with us, should we choose to become bitter. It extends to other relationships and ruins the connection we once had with our sister. Let us learn from Rachel and not take the chance at destroying the relationships we need in our lives.

When we covet, we are essentially telling God what He has given us is not enough. It is a slap in the face to Him. We are informing Him that our peace is not sufficient. Our joy is not abundant. Our relationships are not adequate. Our health is not plentiful. His provision is not enough and, worst of all, His breath of life is not enough. That has to hurt Him as a Father. I am a daddy's girl to the core. My father's love for me and mine for him go beyond anything I could explain. He has made so many sacrifices for our family. He has repeatedly gone without his needs to give us what we want. How could I ever tell him that anything he has done has not been enough? I am sure it would bring him to tears. It would immediately diminish all he has sacrificed for me. That is what we do to God when we display jealousy towards others rather than celebration and genuine joy. Jealously is a thief. It steals the opportunity to celebrate the greatest gifts from God with the people we love. It

We must repent of a

discontented

heart and accept

that His *path* will

lead to our *purpose.*

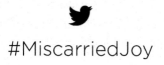

#MiscarriedJoy

displaces our trust in a loving God and is a barrier to reaching our greatest potential in Jesus Christ. When we come to the realization that we can trust God to give us *our sufficient* portion, we will be relieved in the midst of our waiting.

DROWNING DISCONTENTMENT

"First, help me never to tell a lie. Second, give me neither poverty nor riches! Give me just enough to satisfy my needs." (Proverbs 30:8)

Rachel lived a life of discontentment. Oh what a miserable way to live! She wanted everything except what she already had. She wanted Leah's life, Leah's womb and Leah's ability to have so many children. Her life was a perfect example of the disharmony that occurs when you are not happy with what God has provided. If there was another group of people that are known for complaining and never being satisfied, it would have to be the Israelites. I specifically recall them, like us, wanting a specific thing at a specific time.

"Soon the people began to complain about their hardship, and the LORD heard everything they said. Then the LORD's anger blazed against them, and he sent a fire to rage among them, and he destroyed some of the people in the outskirts of the camp...Then the foreign rabble who were traveling with the Israelites began to crave the good things of Egypt. And the people of Israel also began to complain. "Oh, for some meat!" they exclaimed. "We remember the fish we used to eat for free in Egypt. And we had all the cucumbers, melons, leeks, onions, and

*garlic we wanted. But now our appetites are gone. All we
ever see is this manna!" (Numbers 11:1,4-6)*

God had provided more than enough of everything the
Israelites needed. They were so focused on receiving the
food *they* wanted that they were blinded to God's plan. They
disregarded what God was doing for them. I mean He did
set them free and was in the process of transitioning them
to The Promised Land. But none of that mattered in this
moment. They wanted meat instead of manna, though it
would still satisfy their hunger. They were more wrapped up
in what God *wasn't* doing for them. They were more troubled
with their need for physical gratification than the lasting
spiritual fulfillment they would gain from the journey. They
complained and walked in a state of discontentment.

Being content is the supreme acceptance of all that
encompasses your life – your struggles, your pain, your
broken heart, your past, your joy and whatever is in your
future. Contentment should be effortless, but the truth is
that it's arduous. Jesus' crucifixion, death and resurrection
has given us security and freedom from pain and sorrow even
in tribulation and disappointments. He is truly sufficient to
meet all of your needs, dear sister. Dwelling in satisfaction
when you have some real, deep, unmet desires can seem like
an insurmountable task to achieve. I mean how do I have
happiness with heartaches? How can I be expected to practice
patience amongst pressure and pain? How can I be content
when I am confused? Through the help of the Holy Spirit.

*"But the Helper (Comforter, Advocate, Intercessor –
Counselor, Strengthener, Standby), the Holy Spirit,
whom the Father will send in My name [in My place, to*

*represent Me and act on My behalf], He will teach you
all things. And He will help you remember everything
that I have told you." (John 14:26 AMP)*

We rid ourselves of envy only by surrendering our desires
to God so He can satisfy them in His timing. We must
repent of a discontented heart and accept that His path will
lead to our purpose. The lessons modeled through biblical
women shouldn't be implemented because we want a baby,
but because we yearn to be obedient to Jesus Christ; it is Him
we must aim to please. Everything in this world is temporary.
In our spiritual journeys, it is crucial that we set our hearts on
eternal rewards. We must trust God will honor His promises
in our lives. When we become content with what we have, we
yield to God's plan for our lives.

*"Do not love the world or anything in the world. If
anyone loves the world, love for the Father is not in
them. For everything in the world – the lust of the flesh,
the lust of the eyes, and the pride of life – comes not from
the Father but from the world. The world and its desires
pass away, but whoever does the will of God lives forever."
(2 John 2:15-17 NIV)*

When envy is transformed to love *in* us, God can
then work *through* us. Be mindful that *"God is able to bless
you abundantly, so that in all things at all times, having
all that you need, you will abound in every good work"*
(2 Corinthians 9:8 NIV). I want you to take a quick minute
to think about your life overall. Is there more good than bad?
Do you have everything you need? Are you blessed beyond
measure? In spite of all that has happened in your life, hasn't

God kept you, blessed you and provided more than you have asked? Your story is not over. Keep walking. Whenever I feel a spirit of discontentment coming, I pray and read one of my favorite quotes. Quickly quench the spirit of discontentment.

"Happiness cannot be traveled to, owned, earned, worn or consumed. Happiness is a spiritual experience of living every moment with love, grace and gratitude."
(Denis Waitley)

CHAPTER 6

~◦≈◦~

The Waiting Room

"There was a certain man from Ramathaim, a Zuphite from the hill country of Ephraim, whose name was Elkanah son of Jeroham, the son of Elihu, the son of Tohu, the son of Zuph, an Ephraimite. He had two wives; one was called Hannah and the other Peninnah. Peninnah had children, but Hannah had none. Year after year this man went up from his town to worship and sacrifice to the Lord Almighty at Shiloh, where Hophni and Phinehas, the two sons of Eli, were priests of the Lord. Whenever the day came for Elkanah to sacrifice, he would give portions of the meat to his wife Peninnah and to all her sons and daughters. But to Hannah he gave a double portion because he loved her, and the Lord had closed her womb. Because the Lord had closed Hannah's womb, her rival kept provoking her in order to irritate her. This went on year after year. Whenever Hannah went up to the house of the Lord, her rival provoked her till she wept and would not

eat. Her husband Elkanah would say to her, "Hannah,
why are you weeping? Why don't you eat? Why are you
downhearted? Don't I mean more to you than ten sons?"
(1 Samuel 1:5-8 NIV)

When many think of barren women in the bible, Hannah is often the first name that comes to mind. The genealogy verses in the bible are often the ones we skim through or skip over. But there's something powerful to be learned by looking back into Hannah's family tree. She was part of the Jewish nation, which had experienced infertility in previous generations. We are first introduced to her during one of the darkest periods in Israel's history. Israel was in trouble. They were breaking covenant, sin was proliferating and many were turning away from God and towards idols. The quality of leadership was weak. God needed a man who would lead His people back towards the way of righteousness. But before that could happen, He needed a woman who would be willing to raise her son according to His standards *and* dedicate him back to God. Little did Hannah know, she was the woman God needed. Hannah is a well-known woman from the Bible. She is popular, not because of her struggle with infertility, but because of the power and sincerity of her prayers.

Hannah, whose name means favor, was in the fight of her life. She was the favorite wife of Elkanah; Peninnah was the other. Hannah was unable to conceive, while Peninnah had blessed Elkanah with children. Hannah's situation definitely did not seem to communicate God's favor, if you ask me. In fact, it was a sign of social embarrassment to her husband. But because he loved her so much, he remained devoted to her despite the social criticism he was probably receiving. As mentioned in previous chapters, children were very important to society in these times. So important that if a wife could not bear children, it was customary in Middle Eastern culture to give one of her servant girls to her husband to bear children in her place. Polygamy was adopted from a heathen culture. It was never God's will and has never been displayed without the accompanying heartache that comes along with it. Elkanah was a good man, a loving husband to his precious wife. He showed Hannah great favoritism over Peninnah.

"But to Hannah he gave a double portion because he loved her, and the LORD had closed her womb." (1 Samuel 1:5 NIV)

Usually when you have great favor, you also have its companion, hatred. They go hand in hand. Everyone will not be ecstatic about the favor on your life. Elkanah went above and beyond to make Hannah happy. He embraced her barrenness, often validated his love for her and made every attempt to fill the large gaps in her heart. But nothing he attempted was enough for Hannah. Her inability to have a child devastated her and made her feel insignificant. She constantly thought about her failures to have children. I bet she felt great disappointment every month "Aunt Flo" showed up. As if her state of barrenness was not enough, she had to live with a woman who taunted her at every opportunity.

Peninnah hated Hannah. She was cruel and conniving towards her. She tormented poor Hannah day after day and year after year to the point that it made her sick. She was dead set on not letting Hannah forget, even if only for a moment, that she was unable to give Elkanah a son. She constantly provoked her and it caused serious tension in the family. Elkanah did everything he could to build Hannah up while Peninnah did all she could to break Hannah down. She was hateful, heartless, cold-blooded and brutal towards poor Hannah. Yet, our sister had to live with this torture every single day.

Hannah was a very tolerant woman. I mean, can you imagine living with the woman who was able to give your husband the children he desired while you remained childless? How did Hannah feel watching Elkanah interact with his children who did not belong to her? It must have been painful and humiliating. She was a woman with a sorrowful spirit. She was troubled, distressed, grieving, in deep anguish and felt worthless. *"In her deep anguish Hannah prayed to the LORD, weeping bitterly" (1 Samuel 1:10 NIV).* Hannah had a suffering that invaded her entire being. Suffering is not always a consequence of our personal sin. Sometimes, it can be God's perfect will for us. Hannah's suffering was planned by Him. God closed her womb and it was not without purpose. In her desperation, Hannah ran to God. I have found that pain increases our capacity for God. The greater our capacity, the more we are filled with His power to endure.

Hannah had reached the point where emotional support from anyone wasn't enough to ease the pain in her heart. It wasn't that her husband failed to try; his efforts weren't effective. Have you felt that way? I surely have. I would venture to say that I have one of the greatest support systems a woman could ask for. My husband, parents and best friends provide words of encouragement and prayers whenever they feel I need it. But God has allowed each of us to enter into a territory we are powerless to change with our own strength. When we come out of this, we will *know* the great extent of His power. The only way

The *tears* we sow

today are *watering* the

seeds of the *promises*

we will receive tomorrow.

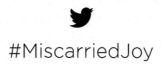

#MiscarriedJoy

Hannah was going to find true fulfillment was by birthing the promise God had given her.

Peninnah was living out her name, which means pearl. *"Natural Pearls form when an irritant - usually a parasite and not the proverbial grain of sand - works its way into an oyster, mussel, or clam. As a defense mechanism, a fluid is used to coat the irritant. Layer upon layer of this coating, called 'nacre', is deposited until a lustrous pearl is formed."[8]* Pearls are beautiful and expensive, but they are formed out of great aggravation. Miss Peninnah was doing a great job with making a pearl out of Hannah! Every day Hannah looked at Peninnah interacting with her children she probably cried, "God something is missing from my life! When are you going to make me a mother?"

Aggravation is often what pushes us to fill the missing voids in our lives. The more frustrated we become, the more we will set our focus on God. But poor Hannah had reached her threshold. She was tired of watching Peninnah have baby after baby. She was tired of being pushed, provoked and persecuted. She was exhausted with being favored but bound in the agony she was experiencing. Like mine and yours, this part of her life just didn't seem fair. She needed deliverance from an intolerable situation. So she gathered up all the strength she had in her, got up from the table and made her way to Shiloh, alone.

> *"Once when they had finished eating and drinking in Shiloh, Hannah stood up. Now Eli the priest was sitting on his chair by the doorpost of the Lord's house. In her deep anguish Hannah prayed to the Lord, weeping bitterly. And she made a vow, saying, "Lord Almighty, if you will only look on your servant's misery and*

remember me, and not forget your servant but give her a son, then I will give him to the Lord for all the days of his life, and no razor will ever be used on his head."

As she kept on praying to the Lord, Eli observed her mouth. Hannah was praying in her heart, and her lips were moving but her voice was not heard. Eli thought she was drunk and said to her, "How long are you going to stay drunk? Put away your wine."

"Not so, my lord," Hannah replied, *"I am* **a woman who is deeply troubled.** *I have not been drinking wine or beer;* **I was pouring out my soul to the Lord.** *Do not take your servant for a wicked woman; I have been* **praying here out of my great anguish and grief."** *(1 Samuel 1:9-16)*

Hannah took her pain, frustration, anguish, grief and sorrow and laid it all on the altar. Every single emotion was left there. She probably told God how much she disliked Peninnah. She probably expressed her weariness and frustration with Him, too. I bet she was brutally honest with God when she met Him at Shiloh. You see, Hannah was well aware that the altar was the place where her burdens would be lifted, her bitterness would be uprooted and her broken heart would be mended. Even if God didn't heal her barrenness, she needed Him to heal her bitterness. She needed a spirit of peace that would help her to thrive while living in such a hostile environment.

Hannah cried and prayed to the point where Eli thought she was drunk. She poured out her soul to the Lord. Though the Lord had shut her womb, her heart was still open to

The *manifestation*

we are hoping for

won't *materialize*

without faith-filled,

zealous petitions.

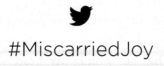

#MiscarriedJoy

Him. She believed God and found refuge from her pain in the sweet presence of her prayers. I know from personal experience this was a challenge to Hannah, because it is for me. Has it been difficult for you to pray in faith when what you have tried to give birth to has been miscarried? Isn't it hard to pray when you feel so spiritually ineffective? Hannah looked beyond her emotions and focused on her needs.

Earlier in the day, Hannah had been so downcast and depressed that she was physically sick. But when she arose from the Altar and left Shiloh, she embodied a new strength. No one could tell the difference from the outside, but she felt relieved and at peace on the inside. She had a transformation in her attitude, her outlook, and a new confidence in God's promise to her. She made it clear to God she was willing to give up what she wanted most to dedicate her life and her son's future to the service of the Lord. When she returned home, she exhibited one of the greatest acts of faith. She rested in God's promise.

As I reflected on the small part of Hannah's life that is told in scripture, I received revelation of her strength, tenacity, maturity and patience. I also learned that postponing the conception and birth of her son was part of God's plan. Her blessing was delayed but it certainly was not denied! So many of us become focused on the external circumstances that we never stop to think about what God is trying to do for us inwardly. Hannah blocked out the taunting, she remained steadfast in her faith and even increased her prayer life. She drowned out all of the noise and went to pray before God.

THE PICTURE OF HER PAIN

I wish I could have been friends with Hannah. We share a similar depth of pain. I know there were times when Hannah felt so alone. Her suffering was terribly personal, just like yours and mine. It affected her worth, her self-esteem and her image as a woman. Oh Hannah, we would have been connected at the hip. She was blessed with favor but it came in very strange places. I mean who really prefers a double portion of something that fails to come close to satisfying your deepest physical and spiritual need?

Elkanah couldn't resolve this issue for her and our husbands cannot erase the pain and emptiness we feel either. Words of encouragement and validation of love just won't do. When tears begin to fall from my eyes in the middle of a conversation about our future or reflections of our past, my husband can wipe the tears, but he may not always be able to feel the desperation and pain in my heart. Our friends and family can sympathize, but until someone has personally felt this pain, they won't truly understand.

Many of us are at different stages of this journey. Maybe you have been unable to conceive for many years. Maybe you are fresh off the loss of your first pregnancy. Maybe you have recently been informed that you won't be able to bear children. Maybe you are considering fertility options. Regardless of where you are in this journey, your pain is real. You have experienced a wide array of emotions and you should not allow anyone to minimize the severity of your hurt. You have been spiritually and emotionally wounded. The enemy has made attempts to steal your promises, your joy, and increase your pain. Like Hannah, we are in a fight. Have you ever had a physical fight? Has anyone ever physically stolen something from you? Have you ever been intimidated by someone you perceived to be bigger or better than you?

We have all probably encountered some type of fight. Today, we are in a spiritual battle. The enemy's attacks may be larger than we have ever anticipated, but he will not be the victor. Ladies, we cannot let him win. During a fight, you become focused solely on the target, your enemy. You hone in on the areas where he or she is weak and that is where you throw your punches. Sometimes they land where you want them and sometimes you miss. But in a spiritual fight, you are more than well-equipped with the armor needed to win. The enemy's strategy is to punch us in the areas of our weakness and to amplify the things God has not yet done in our lives.

Satan wants us to lose hope and trust in the only One who can give life. This experience of wanting yet waiting can be a real struggle. *"For we are not fighting against flesh-and-blood enemies, but against evil rulers and authorities of the unseen world, against mighty powers in this dark world, and against evil spirits in the heavenly places. Therefore, put on every piece of God's armor so you will be able to resist the enemy in the time of evil. Then after the battle you will still be standing firm"* (Ephesians 6:12-13). Never leave your war room without your armor. Put on the breastplate of righteousness, fasten your belt of truth around your waist, stand firm in the peace that comes from God's Word, keep the shield of faith in front of you, and take the helmet of salvation and the sword of the Spirit. Most importantly, *"Pray in the Spirit at all times and on every occasion. Stay alert and be persistent in your prayers for all believers everywhere"* (Ephesians 6:18).

The greater our

capacity for

God, the more

we are *filled* with

His power to *endure.*

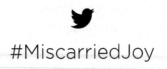

\#MiscarriedJoy

Hannah teaches us a very powerful lesson. She was childless, but she was not void of faith. She lived with a persecutor that pushed her to a posture of prayer and an emptiness that pushed her into the presence of God. Even though Hannah probably had a few friends and a loving husband who worked to mend her brokenness and make her feel accepted and loved, she knew that only God could give her what she desperately desired. She knew Shiloh was the only place where she could trade in her sorrows for joy, her pain for peace and her fears for faith. It was only in the Presence of God and through her trust in Him that her greatest need would be fulfilled. We know a bit about the pain and sorrow she felt, don't we? We too have cried countless tears. But I have great news. *"They that sow in tears shall reap in joy" (Psalm 126:5 KJV)*.

Tears are often our way to express emotions when words just won't do. We cry tears of happiness, joy, sorrow, grief, and emotional or physical pain. *"For everything there is a season, a time for every activity under heaven. A time to cry and a time to laugh" (Ecclesiastes 3:1,4)*. In this season of waiting I have cried for so many different reasons and I am sure you can relate. We have cried as we reflect, cried as we hope for the future, and shed tears of happiness as we see God manifest the baby blessing in the lives of others. It may feel as if God isn't moved by our tears, but He is concerned. He sees the tears we cry in our secret place and He knows our pain. Our Father isn't detached or unsympathetic towards us. Rather, He is there in the passionate cries that communicate our needs, pain, desires and desperation.

"The eyes of the Lord watch over those who do right; his ears are open to their cries for help." (Psalm 34:15)

When Jesus received news of Lazarus' death, he went to Mary and Martha's home. Mary fell at His feet and cried. *"When Jesus saw her weeping and saw the other people wailing with her, a deep anger welled up within him, and he was deeply troubled. 'Where have you put him?' he asked them. They told him, 'Lord, come and see.' Then Jesus wept" (John 11:33-35).* Jesus felt Mary's pain for her brother. He has compassion and sympathy for us, His children. We serve a God who cares and a God who is moved by the faith behind our tears. Psalm 56:8 reminds us that God is deeply concerned with every single detail of our lives and because of his great compassion, He catches *every* tear that is shed.

"You keep track of all my sorrows. You have collected all my tears in your bottle. You have recorded each one in your book."

The tears that we sow today are watering the seeds of the promises we will receive tomorrow. God is using this test to mature us spiritually so that we may become the women others can call upon when situations are bleak, chaos is abounding, and calamity is breaking out. I often wonder what happened to the wailing women from the biblical times. I asked God this same question in my quiet time with Him and He whispered, *"You are becoming one of them."* Remember that Hannah was living in a time when the nation of Israel was in total chaos. As time passed, things got worse and God was preparing to bring judgment on the people in Jerusalem for their disobedience.

"Who is wise enough to understand all this? Who has been instructed by the LORD and can explain it to others?

Why has the land been so ruined that no one dares to travel through it? The LORD replies, "This has happened because my people have abandoned my instructions; they have refused to obey what I said. Instead, they have stubbornly followed their own desires and worshiped the images of Baal, as their ancestors taught them. So now, this is what the LORD of Heaven's Armies, the God of Israel, says: Look! I will feed them with bitterness and give them poison to drink. I will scatter them around the world, in places they and their ancestors never heard of, and even there I will chase them with the sword until I have destroyed them completely." (Jeremiah 9:12-16)

The people of Israel had moved so far away from God and they were in a crisis. But there was help available. God's remedy in the bleak condition of this nation was to call for the wailing women. A wail is a mournful cry full of pain, grief, misery, exasperation and disappointment; it is to truly lament for something or on behalf of someone else. God's response was for the people to wail, or cry out to Him.

"This is what the Lord Almighty says: 'Consider now! Call for the wailing women to come; send for the most skillful of them. Let them come quickly and wail over us till our eye overflow with tears and water streams from our eyelids." (Jeremiah 9:17-18 NIV)

I find it very interesting that God instructed the people to call for the wailing women; the women whom had probably experienced past disappointment and great challenges that pushed their faith to the ultimate test. These were the women who knew how and when to pray. Every situation we experience in our lives should increase the strength and endurance of our faith. The perpetuation of Hannah's hostile environment produced a wailing woman who could move mountains with her prayers. She knew it was necessary to take prayer to the next level. A simple "God, please make this happen for me" just wouldn't do.

Hannah had to get on her face, forget about everything and everyone around her and war in the spirit to bring a change in her life. God wants us to be quick to pour out our spirit before Him and to pray without ceasing (1 Thessalonians 5:17). It is the wailing women who have the passion to call on His promises and stand firm on His Word. God needs wailing women to bring Him into the situation and confess that no weapon formed against us shall prosper. He is developing each of us to become the wailing women He needs. Had Hannah not been tormented, aggravated, and barren, her prayers would not have had the power to change the entire direction of a generation. A woman's supplication can bring blessings to her home, her family, her workplace and, yes, even a nation.

A DESPERATE HEART

There was a time when I prayed simply out of habit. As I grew closer to God, I learned that my prayers were intimate communication with Him. In my prayer time, would hear His leading in my life, His promises to me and receive His comfort when I needed it most. When I started experiencing challenges in my life and communicating with God daily, my prayer life turned from routine into relationship. But now that I am experiencing temporary challenges having children, I have learned the difference between religious prayers and passionate prayers. Although we live in a time where fertility treatments and other technology are available, none of it will be successful without God's divine intervention. Our victory in life is relative to our struggle.

What comes easy to some women is the very same thing for which we must labor in prayer. Is it painful? Absolutely! But I have learned the greater your purpose, the greater your pain. The manifestation we are hoping for won't materialize without faith-filled, zealous petitions. Hannah's prayers are a terrific model for us in our situations. We have to take every feeling and lay it at the altar. Release your hurts, stress and burdens to God.

Hannah yielded the pain of her barrenness through weeping and sincere, heart-felt prayers. Genuine faith motivates us to transfer our circumstances over to God. He will not perform anything on our behalf until we commit our entire being to Him. We must totally let go of what we want and give control to God. Hannah released everything at Shiloh. She never complained to her husband; she prayed to God. I imagine this wasn't the first time she prayed to God for children. It must have been a constant prayer of hers. She was comforted and changed in the place of prayer. She got up with a different perspective on the situation.

We must do the very same thing! Our infertility or miscarried joy may be God's purpose, just as it was for Hannah. He closed Hannah's womb to see what it would produce in her and maybe, just maybe, He is doing the same in our lives. The decisions we make will determine the outcome we receive. What if Hannah decided to abide in self-pity after

Our greatest *needs*

will only be fulfilled

through our time in

the *presence*

of God.

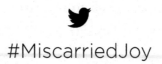

#MiscarriedJoy

discovering she was barren? What would have happened if she remained discouraged, bitter and jealous? Instead of exuding these emotions, her desperation led to prayer, which led to the blessing of reproduction.

Her prayers captured the heart of God. This may be the season in our life that pushes us to desperation. I don't know about you, but I am there – desperate for God to move in this area of my life. Hannah was so desperate that she made a vow to God to relinquish the very thing she was asking for – a son. Oh what a price she paid! Her prayer and the sacrifice she made paid the price for the powerful anointing on Samuel. She didn't just give birth to a son; she gave birth to a king, a prophet and the last of the judges. But she had to give it all up.

"The eyes of the LORD search the whole earth in order to strengthen those whose hearts are fully committed to him." (2 Chronicles 16:9)

God found this kind of heart in his daughter, Hannah. Guess what? He wants to develop that same kind of heart in you and me. Hannah paid a price for her son that very few would be willing to pay. She became abundantly fruitful, but it was birthed out of her barrenness. She later gave birth to three more sons and two daughters. Maybe God still has you in the waiting room because He wants to see if you will become one of those desperate, wailing women. Maybe he needs to develop some areas that will be crucial for parenting. Maybe he is developing your prayer life. Maybe your story will be used to deliver someone else from depression and disappointment. Or maybe He is longing to release another great king on the earth through you, and it isn't the perfect time just yet. Whatever the reason, which may be different for each of us, we must have full confidence in God's sovereignty and control over our lives. Hannah praised God for making her strong, for rescuing her from her test, for being her rock and solid foundation. He is the same for us today. Hannah's prayer in 1 Samuel 2 can serve as a confession of faith while we patiently await God to call us out of the waiting room!

HANNAH'S PRAYER OF PRAISE

¹ Then Hannah prayed:
"My heart rejoices in the LORD!
The LORD has made me strong.
Now I have an answer for my enemies;
I rejoice because you rescued me.
² No one is holy like the LORD!
There is no one besides you;
there is no Rock like our God.

³ "Stop acting so proud and haughty!
Don't speak with such arrogance!
For the LORD is a God who knows what you have done;
he will judge your actions.
⁴ The bow of the mighty is now broken,
and those who stumbled are now strong.
⁵ Those who were well fed are now starving,
and those who were starving are now full.
The childless woman now has seven children,
and the woman with many children wastes away.
⁶ The LORD gives both death and life;
he brings some down to the grave but raises others up.

⁷The LORD makes some poor and others rich;
    he brings some down and lifts others up.
        ⁸He lifts the poor from the dust
    and the needy from the garbage dump.
        He sets them among princes,
            placing them in seats of honor.
        For all the earth is the LORD's,
            and he has set the world in order.

        ⁹"He will protect his faithful ones,
    but the wicked will disappear in darkness.
        No one will succeed by strength alone.
¹⁰Those who fight against the LORD will be shattered.
        He thunders against them from heaven;
            the LORD judges throughout the earth.
        He gives power to his king;
    he increases the strength of his anointed one."

CHAPTER 7

The Perfect Delay

What if? Is that a question you have asked yourself on any stop in this journey? What if the doctor tells me I will never be able to bear children? What if my age is a factor in preventing conception? What if I receive the news my pregnancy will be high risk? What if I am not ovulating? What if I never have any children? *What if.* These are words of doubt that lead your mind down a path to focus on the worst case scenarios. Some of these questions may be your current physical reality, but your solution is not beyond God's spiritual capability. Every woman has a different experience along her journey to motherhood. Some have yet to receive the news of a positive pregnancy, while others have trouble keeping babies in the womb. We are all different ages, ethnicities, and have various genetic makeups that may factor into our ability to conceive or have easy, low-risk pregnancies. Wherever you are in your journey today, I want to encourage you to keep going. Keep believing and keep praying. I know what you may be thinking. It's easy to say but so hard to do.

"Keep the faith!" is an expression you've probably heard many times throughout this journey to becoming a mom. I know I have, and it usually comes from someone that has no emotional understanding of what I am experiencing. My reply often is, *"I know that God is going to do it,"* but my mind is wondering, *"God, when are You going to do it for me?"* As I stated in a previous chapter, my husband and I have been trying for almost two years to have a baby and while that may not seem like a long time to some, it has been the greatest test of my faith. But I know there are women reading this book who have been trying for years to have a baby and are still waiting. There are also women who have been informed of a physical or medical condition that is preventing pregnancy from occurring in your body. What a great test of faith and the perfect backdrop for a miracle to take place in your life! You, my sister, are blessed to have God use you to get glory and to inspire others to believe only in Him. Not everyone has the opportunity to be used in such an extraordinary manner.

Earlier, I shared that my mom was told she would never be able to have children years after giving birth to me. I have permission to share a bit of her story with you. My mother experienced a miscarriage when I was ten years old. It was devastating to her and scary to me. Just as mothers have an unexplainable love for their children, we, too, have an intense love for our parents. But there is something special about the relationship we have with moms. I mean, they did give birth to us. We call for them when we are happy, sad, rejoicing or in pain. So imagine watching your mother go through the stages of miscarriage – pain, disappointment, agony, and hurt – without being able to help her. There was nothing I could do. When she cried, I cried all the more. It was not a happy day in the Jones household. This incident left a hole in each of our hearts. The brother or sister I thought I was having was now in heaven with Jesus. The comforting words from others didn't diminish the pain we felt. As time passed, our hearts healed. But there was definitely an immense amount of love that we yearned to give to another person.

Shortly after the miscarriage, my mom experienced an ectopic pregnancy that caused one of her fallopian tubes to burst. It required removal of her entire tube and left her with a much lower chance of getting pregnant. In fact, the doctors told her that it would be near impossible. My parents then considered adoption, but we depended more on our prayers for God to do the impossible. God performed a miracle in our lives! At five weeks pregnant, my mom received news that God had doubly blessed her with twin girls! He performed what the "experts" deemed impossible. He is just that kind of God! As a little girl I knew *about* God, but me praying for my sisters gave me the opportunity to *know* God and taught me that He is the God that hears my prayers and delights in answering them.

GOD DELIGHTS IN MIRACLES

Physical limitations do not limit or intimidate God. He can and will do miraculous things through anyone that makes themselves available to Him. Consider what he did for Zechariah and Elizabeth.

"When Herod was king of Judea, there was a Jewish priest named Zechariah. He was a member of the priestly order of Abijah, and his wife, Elizabeth, was also from the priestly line of Aaron. Zechariah and

Physical

limitations

do not limit or

intimidate God.

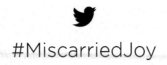

#MiscarriedJoy

Elizabeth were righteous in God's eyes, careful to obey all of the Lord's commandments and regulations. They had no children because Elizabeth was unable to conceive, and they were both very old. While Zechariah was in the sanctuary, an angel of the Lord appeared to him, standing to the right of the incense altar. Zechariah was shaken and overwhelmed with fear when he saw him. But the angel said, "Don't be afraid, Zechariah! God has heard your prayer. Your wife, Elizabeth, will give you a son, and you are to name him John. You will have great joy and gladness, and many will rejoice at his birth, for he will be great in the eyes of the Lord." (Luke 1:5-6, 11-15a)

Zechariah – whose name means "The Lord remembers"[9] – was a very old Jewish priest. He was married to Elizabeth – whose name means "my God is an oath."[10] They loved God whole-heartedly, obeyed all of His commandments and committed to a lifestyle of holiness. They were *"upright in the sight of God."* While many of our problems in life are a direct result of our sin, there are some challenges that God allows for the sole purpose of growing in our love for and obedience to Him. This was the case for the love birds, Zechariah and Elizabeth. God had a special plan for their lives that was beyond anything they could visualize. They were happily married but had a huge emptiness in their hearts. Elizabeth was barren and they were both well beyond child-bearing age. They were in what some would call a hopeless situation.

Zechariah committed his problem to God through prayer. Although his request for a child remained unanswered, he continued to serve and do the work God had called him to do. In the midst of working, an angel of God appeared to inform him that God had heard his prayers and Elizabeth would give birth to a son whom they would name John. Zechariah was the first person in four-hundred years recorded in scripture to receive a direct word from God. I love how God showed up in the most unexpected moment in the midst of his serving. I don't know of too many women who don't yearn to become mothers. Yet when one of our greatest desires becomes one of our toughest challenges, we can easily become disheartened and discouraged. It is easier to quit rather than keep going. It is so easy to focus on the problem rather than give greater attention to the blessings we are experiencing in the present. Zechariah and Elizabeth chose to focus on blessings over barrenness.

Robin Sharma, a world-renowned leadership speaker, once gave some powerful advice which I think is helpful for us to remember in any season of waiting. He said, *"What you focus on grows, what you think about expands, and what you dwell upon determines your destiny."*[11] We must stop focusing on the fact that God has not yet blessed us with the children we desire and focus on what He has already done in our lives and what He is able to do.

Lake Michigan is my favorite place of serenity in the summer time. I love to sit and reflect on God's beautiful creation and His awesome wonder that is before us every day. My husband and I were once downtown Chicago and decided to have a romantic walk along the lake. I turned to him and said, "Babe, you can't see where the lake ends. I know that it ends somewhere but I cannot see it from here." To which he replied, *"The only way to get to the end of the lake is to get in the boat and just keep going."* We often wonder when this part of our journey to motherhood will commence. But we will never know if we quit.

Zechariah and Elizabeth probably didn't stop praying, and the problem wasn't where they chose to concentrate. I personally know this advice is definitely easier said than done. Every time I hold a baby or receive the news of a coming bundle of joy, I think about when my precious bundles of joy will arrive. But that cannot be my focus daily, because I have work to do in the Kingdom of God. This challenge is just a minor obstacle that will become a large part of the fulfillment of my purpose for the glory of God. And it will be the same for you, too!

Luke 1 doesn't share much about Elizabeth's desire for a child. But because she is a woman built with nurturing characteristics, we can gather that being childless and up in age was a painful experience that left her feeling unfulfilled and lonely. But we do know that she still remained faithful to God. Oh the joy she must have felt when Zechariah came home with the news they would be parents. She was probably a bit confused too, given that he was physically speechless! After the angel Gabriel delivered this word from God, Zechariah doubted the promise.

> "Zechariah said to the angel, "How can I be sure this will happen? I'm an old man now, and my wife is also well along in years. Then the angel said, "I am Gabriel! I stand in the very presence of God. It was he who sent me to bring you this good news! But now, since you didn't believe what I said, you will be silent and unable to speak until the child is born. For my words will certainly be fulfilled at the proper time." (Luke 1:18-20)

There are consequences to doubting the promises of God. Elizabeth, on the other hand, showed no doubts about

God's divine ability to fulfill His promise to them. Soon after receiving the news, she became pregnant. She knew her son was a long-hoped for gift from God.

What if they would have quit praying once they were well-beyond the age of safe child-bearing? What if you stop praying because the doctors, who have no power over God, informed you that you may never have a child for various reasons? Have you received less than favorable news and forgotten about the God who specializes in miracles? You must not allow your physical conditions to blur your spiritual confidence in what God is able to perform.

Don't stop praying and standing in faith because your situation *seems* hopeless. God delights in performing the impossible and nothing is too hard for Him. Don't run from this difficult circumstance. Stay in the boat to see where your Lake Michigan ends. Running will only compound the problem because God will not be able to develop your spiritual tenacity if you run. Grow through it! Maybe you think the Lord has forgotten about you, but He has not. Daily, God is performing the impossible in the lives of His people. Your time is coming. Don't succumb to the pressure and don't fret about this burden. Just keep believing God and keep confessing His word over your situation. Keep serving and keep waiting with a patient expectation for Him to do what he did for Elizabeth for you. He loves you just the same.

A CHILD WITH A PURPOSE

The more I reflect on and study the story of Zechariah and Elizabeth, the more I realize that God's timing is never a delay for Him. It is a delay for us because we often have our own agendas, our own plans and our own timing.

God doesn't *work* according to

our time. He works according to

when we are *ready* to receive

the *blessing*

He has *stored up* for us.

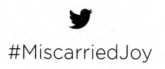

#MiscarriedJoy

Often, we neglect to consult God to ensure our desires match up with His perfect will. It was not by chance that Zechariah was chosen to enter into the holy place on that specific day. It was not by chance they both were very old and without a child. God was actually guiding the events of history to prepare the way for Jesus Christ to come to the earth. And he chose Zechariah and Elizabeth to play an important role in the greatest moment in Christian history. What a privilege! John's purpose was chosen before he was even conceived.

> *"For he will be great in the eyes of the Lord. He must never touch wine or other alcoholic drinks. He will be filled with the Holy Spirit, even before his birth. And he will turn many Israelites to the Lord their God. He will be a man with the spirit and power of Elijah. He will prepare the people for the coming of the Lord. He will turn the hearts of the fathers to their children, and he will cause those who are rebellious to accept the wisdom of the godly." (Luke 1:15-17)*

God knew he had to be set apart in order to effectively walk in his calling. John is the perfect picture of God working through what many deemed impossible – old age and barrenness – to bring about the fulfillment of the prophecies concerning the Messiah, Jesus Christ. *"Look! I am sending my messenger, and he will prepare the way before me. Then the Lord you are seeking will suddenly come to his Temple. The messenger of the covenant, whom you look for so eagerly, is surely coming,"* says the Lord of Heaven's Armies" (Malachi 3:1).John, the manifestation of this prophecy, was going to lead the way. God knew Elizabeth and Zechariah would be the parents of

John the Baptist, yet they had no idea. God also knew when He was going to bring Jesus to the earth and offer the free gift of salvation to the world. What was a delay to Elizabeth, was the perfect timing for God. He is strategic in everything He does. Nothing just happens.

What if your child's purpose is a pivotal key to God's future plans in the earth? Had John been born even a year earlier, he may not have been chosen to prepare the way for Jesus. Paul said, *"But my life is worth nothing to me unless I use it for finishing the work assigned me by the Lord Jesus – the work of telling others the Good News about the wonderful grace of God" (Act 20:24).* Each of us were placed on earth with an assignment. In order for our purpose to be fulfilled, we have to first be available to God and our timing has to be perfectly aligned with His. It is the same with the children that God will birth through us. They are assigned a purpose before they are conceived. We don't have any control over when God chooses to bring them to the earth, but we do have an assignment to pray for them, even before they are born.

"Listen to me, all you in distant lands! Pay attention, you who are far away. The LORD called me before my birth; from within the womb he called me by name." (Isaiah 49:1)

We have partnered in prayer with a few trusted people as we believe God for our children. I encourage you to do the same. But one thing that we had not done until recently is to begin praying for our children and the specific purposes that God will place on their lives. Since God already knows who they will become and what need they will fulfill in the earth, we have been commissioned to pray for the impact they will have on the world and pray against any attacks the enemy would attempt in their lives. Luke 1 records Elizabeth and her cousin Mary, the mother of Jesus, praying over the sons in their wombs. They knew God had great plans for John and Jesus before they were conceived. They glorified God for the transformational impact they would have in the world. It is never too early to start praying for our children. God knows them before they are born.

> *"You made all the delicate, inner parts of my body and knit me together in my mother's womb. Thank you for making me so wonderfully complex! Your workmanship is marvelous — how well I know it. You watched me as I was being formed in utter seclusion, as I was woven together in the dark of the womb.* **You saw me before I was born.** *Every day of my life was recorded in your book. Every moment was laid out before a single day had passed." (Psalm 139:13-16)*

PRAY FOR YOUR UNBORN CHILDREN

"Any concern too small to be turned into a prayer is too small to be made into a burden." (Corrie Ten Boom)

The children you yearn for are on your heart. Anything that stays on our hearts should be brought to God in prayer. Waiting can make us anxious, but the Bible tells us, *"Do not be anxious about anything, but in every situation, by prayer and petition, with thanksgiving, present your requests to God" (Philippians 4:6 NIV).* While Elizabeth and Zechariah are not mentioned again after the birth of John the Baptist, they left a strong legacy of faith for us to believe in The God who achieves the impossible in our lives and in the earth.

Anything that

stays on our

hearts should be

brought to

God in *prayer.*

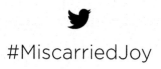

#MiscarriedJoy

As we stand in faith together for God to bless each of us with the children we long for, we must partner our faith with our prayers. As we pray for our children, God will divinely connect us to the purpose He has placed in them. Elizabeth was filled with the Holy Spirit through her son (Luke 1:42).

Zechariah's encounter with Gabriel left him with a new awareness of the greatness of our God and a stronger sense of faith. Because he knew without a doubt (that is faith) that his son would soon be conceived, Elizabeth and Zechariah, even in his inability to speak, probably spent time praying for their son. Our prayers prepare the way for the coming of our children in a similar way that John was leading the way for Jesus (Matthew 3). We don't have to meet our children on earth before we begin specifically praying for them. We should start now. Here are some specific areas that we should be praying for:

- Pray they will be healthy and void of illnesses (3 John 1:2).
- Pray they come to faith at a very early age (Romans 10:17).
- Pray they will trust God completely (Jeremiah 17:7-8).
- Pray your child will love God and delight in obeying His commandments (Deuteronomy 6:5, Matthew 22:37).
- Pray they will desire to know God more and more each day (1 John 4:6-7).
- Pray they will sense God's plan for their lives and accept it at an early age (Ephesians 2:10).
- Pray they will earnestly seek wisdom, discernment and understanding (James 1:5).

- Pray their attention would be focused on doing what is right (Romans 16:19, Proverbs 4:25).
- Pray they will remain in God's truth throughout their lives (Psalm 119:1-3).
- Pray their character would align with God's & that the fruits of the spirit would be evident in their lives (1 John 4:8, Galatians 5:22).
- Pray they will live a life of integrity (Proverbs 11:3, 1 Peter 3:16).
- Pray that God would direct their steps and keep them from falling (Psalm 17:5, Psalm 37:2-34).
- Pray their faith will be strengthened and that they will not have a quitting spirit (Philippians 4:13).
- Pray they will be diligent in their work and that their hand would not be idle (Colossians 3:17).

Your desire may seem delayed, but remember your children must come at the appointed time for their appointed purpose in the earth and in The Kingdom of God. Knowing about Mary's pregnancy must have made Elizabeth be in awe of God's timing. She was the first woman after Mary to hear of the coming Savior. Everything was perfectly planned and excellently executed in God's timing. God goes to great lengths to strengthen our faith, and the ending of your story will be used to help someone witness an amazing act of God.

God doesn't work according to our time. He works according to when we are ready for the blessing He has stored up for us. The natural part of us worries about time, while God is saying, *if you just take up your cross and follow the road that I have paved for you, time wouldn't be a factor to you either.* I encourage you to stop focusing on the fact that you have asked God to bless you with a baby but it hasn't happened *yet*. It doesn't mean God is denying your request; it could mean He is waiting on us to surrender to His purpose and plan – completely! We must completely give everything over to God, live according to His Word, trust His plan and wait on His promises.

> *"I have been young, and now am old; Yet I have not seen the righteous forsaken, nor his descendants begging bread." (Psalm 37:25)*

God has not forgotten about us. Let's get beyond God blessing us and worship Him for who He is. Once we have allowed God to complete the spiritual circumcision in our lives, His promises will follow.

Part Three

Walking in Extraordinary Faith

CHAPTER 8

Labor and Delivery

Sarah. Rachel. Rebekah. Hannah. Elizabeth. You. Me. We are women who have experienced an immense amount of pain and disappointment. In the previous chapters, we took an extensive journey through the lives of these barren women. We witnessed many ways they exhibited great faith, and also actions that had the potential to block the manifestation of God's promises in their lives. We felt their pain, their heartache, the disenchantment and exhaustion from wanting, yet waiting. We were able to empathize with them because, in some way, we are similar to them. I pray that you now have a deeper understanding behind the purpose of your pain. God is doing something to you to get something through you. He is leading us through the wilderness into Canaan, The Promised Land. Not one bit of it feels pleasant, but it will all work out for our good.

I talked to a woman who shared this with me: "I want a baby more than any other physical thing in this world. I think about it every day. It consumes me. When I see other mothers with their babies, I get jealous, run into a secluded space and cry until there are no tears left to fall from my eyes. I am truly blessed; I know that to be true, but I just feel so empty. I hope there is hope left for me, but the doctors fail to think so. What do I do? Why did God choose *me* to experience this?"

Her words left me with an unexplainable sense of compassion. You see, this was a woman who had no idea about what I am experiencing. She was unaware that I felt her pain to the core. I not only heard her heart; her heart and mine were perfectly synchronized. Why is *this* the wilderness God chose for us to bear? Why couldn't it be something that didn't make us feel less than the women we were created to be? The pure sentiment she expressed is probably very similar to yours. But what if we need to finally take the pill from the bottle and swallow the acceptance that this wilderness experience is God's perfectly planned will for our lives?

I know it is tough to hear. I understand there may be moments when you see God as cruel instead of loving. When we read the story of the Israelites' journey into the Promised Land, questioning why it took them forty years to complete an eleven-day journey is effortless. That is, until we are walking in the spiritual shoes they once wore. *"Why did they constantly murmur and complain? Why did they doubt God? If only they had been obedient, they would not have died in the wilderness, but would have inhabited the Promised Land."* It is so easy to recognize their faults and wonder about the whys behind their actions. But now that we are having our own

Sometimes

what we need is

not a change in our

circumstances,

but a change in

our *mindset.*

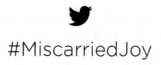

#MiscarriedJoy

wilderness experience, do we demonstrate similar actions that we deemed deplorable? The dust from the blowing wind in the wilderness seems to cloud our eyes doesn't it? Now, our simple belief in God doesn't quite feel like enough to live on. It is almost impossible to not turn our heads towards heaven and screech from the deepest depth of our lungs, *"God, why me?"*

I was taught you should never question God, but, frankly, I think God is fine with us asking why. The prophet Habakkuk did. *"Your eyes are too pure to look on evil; you cannot tolerate wrongdoing. Why then do you tolerate the treacherous? Why are you silent while the wicked swallow up those more righteous than themselves?" (Habakkuk 1:3 NIV).* Jeremiah even attempted to reconcile what he understood about God with what he was witnessing. *"You, LORD, reign forever; your throne endures from generation to generation. Why do you always forget us? Why do you forsake us so long?" (Lamentations 5:19-20 NIV).*

Are you still asking God and yourself the "why me" question? I did for a long time and in total transparency, I still do. But the lives of Sarah, Rebekah, Rachel, Hannah and Elizabeth have made it quite clear that I won't know the answer until I am out of the wilderness. I won't understand all that God is trying to do through me until His work in this area of my life is completed. Hannah didn't know that she was giving birth to a king. Elizabeth was unaware her son would lead the way for Jesus, and Sarah didn't even get to see the great blessing her son had on all of humanity. But they were open and available to be used as His vessels for His glory. The Israelites really got to know God through their time in the wilderness, and so will we. If it pains you to think

God is allowing you to travel through a rough season just so you can know Him better, consider the alternative.

When Pharaoh finally let the people go, God did not lead them along the main road that runs through Philistine territory, even though that was the shortest route to the Promised Land. God said, "If the people are faced with a battle, they might change their minds and return to Egypt." So God led them in a roundabout way through the wilderness toward the Red Sea. Thus the Israelites left Egypt like an army ready for battle." (Exodus 13:17-18)

God doesn't always work in the way we expect Him or in a way that is comfortable for us. He took the Israelites down a path that would take longer, but it was to avoid a danger they had no idea was present. In essence, God was actually protecting them. God knew the other path was full of dangerous, maybe even lethal, encounters. Their experience through the wilderness was for a spiritual purpose and personal protection. God has called us out of Egypt into Canaan to achieve an intimacy that can only be developed through our tenacity to endure. Our character is being developed as we travel through the dry, dusty grounds of the desert. It is here where we will obtain spiritual intimacy, discernment, and direction from our Creator, the King of Kings. It is here where we will experience a profound level of trust and cultivate a confidence in God that He will not allow us to be pushed, pressed or provoked beyond what we are able to tolerate (1 Corinthians 10:13). Don't rush the wilderness journey or bid it away. God is preparing each of us to enter into the land flowing with milk and honey. And when we walk out of this

This season of

waiting

was purposed to

humble us,

not to humiliate us.

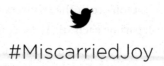

#MiscarriedJoy

waiting season, we will enter into an abundance beyond what we could have ever imagined. We will receive the fullness of joy with a grateful heart.

LABOR PAINS

The moment a woman finds out she is pregnant, there is immense joy, excitement and anticipation. Nine months later, a beautiful bundle of joy will be delivered into the world. What she rarely considers is the time and experiences between the positive pregnancy test and the skin-to-skin contact that will occur between mom and baby. In the fifth week of my second pregnancy, I had evening sickness. Every. Single. Day! It was awful and quickly took my focus off the coming bundle of joy and onto a strategy to get relief or strength to put up with the discomfort. The headaches, fatigue, and malodorous smells were not welcomed, although I knew the end would be marvelous. The Israelites had a similar situation.

> "GOD said, 'I've taken a good, long look at the affliction of my people in Egypt. I've heard their cries for deliverance from their slave masters; I know all about their pain. And now I have come down to help them, pry them loose from the grip of Egypt, get them out of that country and bring them to a good land with wide-open spaces, a land lush with milk and honey, the land of the Canaanite, the Hittite, the Amorite, the Perizzite, the Hivite, and the Jebusite." (Exodus 3:7-8 MSG)

What excitement they must have felt! It was time to leave the land of bondage and enter into a land of freedom. So they followed the instructions and they moved. But they had no idea what was ahead of them. The Israelites were not far from Egypt before they encountered trouble. The Lord said to Moses, *"Tell the Israelites to turn around and make camp at Pi Hahiroth, between Migdol and the sea. Camp on the shore of the sea opposite Baal Zephon. "Pharaoh will think, 'The Israelites are lost; they're confused. The wilderness has closed in on them.' Then I'll make Pharaoh's heart stubborn again and he'll chase after them. And I'll use Pharaoh and his army to put my Glory on display. Then the Egyptians will realize that I am GOD." And that's what happened" (Exodus 14:1-5 MSG).* To Pharaoh, they were in the perfect location for him to attack and they had nowhere to turn. They were certain they were going to die in this seemingly impossible situation.

> *"And they said to Moses, "Why did you bring us out here to die in the wilderness? Weren't there enough graves for us in Egypt? What have you done to us? Why did you make us leave Egypt? Didn't we tell you this would happen while we were still in Egypt? We said, 'Leave us alone! Let us be slaves to the Egyptians. It's better to be a slave in Egypt than a corpse in the wilderness!'" But Moses told the people, "Don't be afraid. Just stand still and watch the LORD rescue you today. The Egyptians you see today will never be seen again. The LORD himself will fight for you. Just stay calm." (Exodus 14:11-12)*

And the Lord did what Moses ensured them. He provided a path of rescue by parting the Red Sea. God did not send them into the wilderness to die, and He has not allowed this waiting journey to destroy our hope. This is probably not the first spiritual obstacle you have encountered in your life, though it may seem like the biggest. God strategically placed

Wilderness

experiences

often come on the

heels of a great

spiritual

breakthrough.

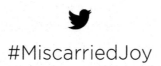

#MiscarriedJoy

the Israelites on the shore of the sea so He could perform a miracle to serve as a reminder of what He can do when all hope is gone. I believe that is what He is doing for me and for you. He wants us in a place where the only available way out is a miraculous move of God on our behalf. Our Red Sea experiences don't exist to aggravate us; rather, to impart expectancy and enthusiasm for what God is preparing to do. Along the road, there will be challenges, but it will make us appreciate the blessing all the more.

A contraction is often the first physical sign of labor. When a woman is in labor, she produces blood, sweat and tears. She has anxiously anticipated this moment for the past nine months, but there is not much that can prepare her for the labor experience. She can think of the stories she has heard from others, she can devise a plan to ease the pain and create a calm environment, but she must still expect the unexpected. Not much will go according to her plan. For her to have the best experience possible, she has to relinquish control and allow the doctors, nurses and even her husband to do what they must to execute a safe delivery. The best thing for her to do is to trust God and push through it. The contractions are going to come and go while getting stronger each time. She cannot predict the pain. And in order for her labor to commence into the delivery of her precious baby, she has to keep going. She cannot press pause, she cannot quit. The process of labor speeds up if you keep moving between the contractions.

I liken the labor experience to that of the Israelites' trip to Canaan. Their journey was filled with insurmountable plagues, attacks and challenges. They did too much complaining and not enough trusting, even with their knowledge of inheriting a land flowing with prosperity. They forgot all that God had previously done in their lives and faltered in their faith. They quickly caught amnesia regarding God's protection from the frogs, gnats, flies, livestock, boils, hail, locust, darkness and being spared from the deaths of their firstborn. God had built a track record of coming through in the clutch. But still, they doubted.

This is a familiar response among women praying to become a mom or living in fear of losing another child. We cry, complain, fail to believe that our dreams will come to pass, and are often tempted to just throw the towel in the fire. We tend to forget the miracles God has performed in our lives and in the lives of others. Trust me, I know what it is like to believe one thing while experiencing the complete opposite; to confess you serve a supernatural God, but still lack a supernatural intervention. Even when it seems as if the walls are closing in and you have no hope left to hold on to, God's hand of love, guidance and protection are there.

He is able to brighten our hearts with inexpressible joy and to bless us with every spiritual blessing in the heavenly realms. In love. In joy. In peace. In pain. In prosperity. All because we are united with Him. God is not withholding your blessing because he is stingy. That is definitely not the God we serve. He delights in pleasing us. He is waiting enthusiastically to give us more than we could ask or think. But to get there, we have to tear down the boundaries that prevent us from experiencing the fullness of an abundant relationship with our Lord and Savior.

"You love him even though you have never seen him. Though you do not see him now, you trust him; and you rejoice with a glorious, inexpressible joy." (1 Peter 1:8)

Huge *struggles*

put you in a perfect

position to *witness*

God give you huge

solutions.

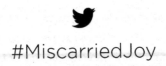

#MiscarriedJoy

Surviving the Wilderness

I cannot wait to become a mom. Now that I have experienced the loss of three children, I am ready and willing to welcome whatever comes along with the pregnancy journey. I don't want the morning sickness, the heartburn, the fatigue, or adverse symptoms of being with child. But if that is what it takes to get to the delivery of my baby, bring it on! I will sacrifice anything I need to ensure that our children get all they need to arrive on this earth healthy and stress-free. But prior to my first pregnancy, I remember sharing with friends that I did not look forward to any of those things during pregnancy. I complained before I even made it to the wilderness. Sometimes what we need is not a change in our circumstances, but a change in our mindset. Why did God make wilderness places? Because without them it would be difficult for us to appreciate the beauty of the multi-colored trees, bright green pastures, and flowing rivers and streams. God also knew that the wilderness would be the perfect place to test his children and help them discover true faith and develop survival skills.

There is a large amount of wilderness in and around Israel. It would be mighty difficult to travel from Egypt to the Promised Land without passing through the wilderness. *"Normally it takes only eleven days to travel from Mount Sinai to Kadesh-barnea, going by way of Mount Seir. But forty years after the Israelites left Egypt, on the first day of the eleventh month, Moses addressed the people of Israel, telling them everything the Lord had commanded him to say"* (Deuteronomy 1:2). It took the children of Israel forty years to make the journey. They got stuck in the wilderness, not just because of their doubt and unbelief, but also because God needed to teach them a few things before inhabiting The Promised Land.

The wilderness is a very common test of our faith. There are rules to successfully survive the journey. We don't want to spiritually die like some of the others. I want to be like Joshua and Caleb. I want to make it through and I want to see you on the other side as well. First, we must comprehend that this season of waiting was purposed to humble us, not to humiliate us. God wants to strip away all pride, selfishness, doubt, and complaining, and get us to the place where we can show gratitude to Him despite our circumstances. It will reveal our level of commitment in obedience to God.

After losing our twins, I felt that I could emotionally heal on my own. Put on the big girl panties and keep it moving, girl! Pick up your face, dry your tears and move on to the next thing in your life. But this wilderness season has been a constant reminder to me that I am not as independent and strong as I like to think. I have to drop my pride and rely totally on Jesus to do what only He can do. This goes beyond Him blessing us with children. This is about Him transforming me from the inside out so that even if I never get all that I want, He is all that I need.

I surely did not expect that I would experience such pain coming off such an exciting time in our lives. I mean isn't the first year of marriage supposed to be pure bliss? As I studied God's Word, I uncovered a compelling, encouraging fact. Wilderness experiences often come on the heels of a great spiritual breakthrough. The children of Israel had just been delivered through the Red Sea so they could escape Pharaoh, and then wandered in the wilderness. Abraham had received a promise, but still had a barren wife. Jesus was baptized and clearly heard the voice of God speaking to Him from heaven right before he was led into the desert and tempted for forty days and forty nights (Matthew 3:16-17). As soon as you come down from the mountain top or receive a promise from God, expect for the enemy to discourage you.

We must not neglect our time with Him. It is crucial that rather than seeking a way out of this circumstance, we daily seek our way into God's presence. In order to remain in perfect peace in the midst of this storm, we must reach out to Him passionately, fervently and consistently. There will never be a day when we are not in need of His love, concern, provision and grace. Daily time with God is a top priority in my life. In that time, I am not bugging Him about when I will have a baby, but I am focused on what His purpose is for me in this season. *God, what do you want me to do for You? How can I grow Your Kingdom?* We must remove the focus off of the Promised Land and onto the Promise Giver.

God is revealing the intention in our hearts. Will you whole-heartedly serve and obey Him even when He allows incredible pain in your life? Will you honor Him? Will you listen to His voice and allow His plan to unfold without your help? My doctor informed me that if I was not pregnant within six months, she wanted me to come into the office for genetic and fertility tests. She wanted to see if she could identify the problem. I initially declined the tests because I know without one shadow of doubt that God has to provide this blessing. Now I am not against testing and other fertility treatments, but God told me that we have to trust Him totally. I believe He will do it and I am going to be obedient to his instructions. I would only cause myself greater stress by being aware of an issue that only God can fix anyhow. God needs us to move from knowing the Word to living the Word. Our hearts and minds are being molded into what God wants it to reflect – His image.

"To everything there is a season, a time for every purpose under heaven." (Ecclesiastes 3:1 NKJV)

So what is the purpose of this desert season? What can the wilderness do for me and for you? It gives us the endurance and strength for success. It opens the door for God to show His supernatural power in your life. In our experiences. In our emotions. And yes, even in our emptiness. After this is over, you will be rugged, tough and stronger in your faith. You will have the ability to persevere. Joshua and Caleb were the survivors of the forty-year journey. Joshua's leadership required a level of spiritual maturity and resolve to guide the people into the land and to gain the victory over their enemies. Caleb, at the ripe old age of eighty-five, was able to drive out the giants and demonic forces that took up residence in Hebron for centuries. David knew about the wilderness. The book of Psalms was written as a result of his sufferings. Jesus began His ministry in Galilee immediately after leaving the wilderness.

Not only does the wilderness develop our character, it breeds humility. When God was done dealing with Moses in the wilderness, he became the humblest man on earth. God does mighty works in the wilderness. He desires to break us down in the same manner.

"Now Moses was very humble – more humble than any other person on earth." (Numbers 12:3)

Gosh, the wilderness can be such a lonely place. I want to escape it, but I know staying here is the best thing for me.

We have to show God that our faith is genuine. We will come out as pure gold after this fire is snuffed.

"*So be truly glad. There is wonderful joy ahead, even though you must endure many trials for a little while. These trials will show that your faith is genuine. It is being tested as fire tests and purifies gold – though your faith is far more precious than mere gold. So when your faith remains strong through many trials, it will bring you much praise and glory and honor on the day when Jesus Christ is revealed to the whole world."*
(1 Peter 1:6-7)

Huge struggles put you in a perfect position to witness God give you huge solutions. Let's not allow these difficulties to turn us away from trusting the God who cares, the God who loves us, and the God who is waiting on the very edge of His heavenly seat to bless our socks off! The wilderness, though unattractive, is precious. This will be one of the biggest blessings in your life and in mine. It will strengthen our witness to others, and will deeply affect the way we relate and minster to God's beloved children – the women who will need encouragement through our story.

I know you may have done all you know to do. You may have even prayed all you know to pray. You have stood on countless promises and still, nothing. I know. I feel your pain. But there is an end to the wilderness. I know you may struggle between God's ability to change these very hard things and his willingness to change them for you. It will work out in the course of time as it did for Sarah, Rebekah, Rachel, Hannah and Elizabeth. So this is what we need to do.

Welcome the hard places.
Start expecting miracles.
Anticipate your breakthrough.
Believe everything you've heard about God.
Keep walking through the fire.
Keep serving through the flood.
Keep living for God.
Keep pushing through the pain.
Keep praying for the manifestation.

God is going to do it for you. You are almost there. Can't you see the Promised Land? I do, and I don't want you to die in the wilderness, so let's walk through this together.

CHAPTER 9

We Are Expecting

"God didn't promise days without pain, laughter without sorrow, or sun without rain, but He did promise strength for the day, comfort for the tears, and light for the day. If God brings you to it, He will bring you through it."
(~Unknown)

Faith – the hopeful expectation that what you are hoping for will manifest although you can't quite see it yet. It is the ability to trust and believe that all is well, although your circumstances say otherwise. It is what Abraham, Isaac, Jacob, Moses and many others stood upon in the face of mere opposition. It is what is necessary for me and for you to get from where we are today to where we want to be tomorrow. As I mentioned before, faith is the currency of the Kingdom. In the world, money buys us what we need or desire. But as citizens of the Kingdom, faith is what we use to get all that we need. Faith is the answer to every problem you encounter. It is the strategy to go from the wilderness to the Promised

Land, from the prison to the palace, and from the flood to the ark. As children of God, we cannot live or be successful without faith. It isn't always easy to operate in it when you have arrived at your divine appointment with disappointment.

"God, you have me in the wilderness, but how long do I have to journey here? I know You have equipped me with survival skills, but God, oh God, how long do I need to use them here? When am I coming out of this?" Maybe you haven't asked God this, but I surely have. I mean, have you ever dreaded going somewhere? You know, that corporate function where you really don't want to work the room? The party with people you don't care to interact with? Or jury duty? When you serve on jury duty, there are specific occurrences that must happen, like the opening statements, the testimonies of the many witnesses, and the back and forth deliberations of the jury. Some cases are open and shut, while others have the tendency to drag far beyond the time you wish to stay. I know you want to run away from this, but where are you going to run to? We don't have the authority to end this waiting season according to our timetable. You cannot control the ending, but you can make the best of it while you're there. This will require a shift in our mindsets.

When I think about waiting, I am often reminded of David. About fifteen years passed between the time he was privately anointed and the time he publicly ruled as king. Imagine being promoted at work with no effective start date. Imagine being engaged with no set wedding date. Think about receiving news that you have won millions of dollars, but you have no idea when you will receive it. Quite frustrating, right? I think that must be how David felt at one point or another. He spent a lot of time waiting for something he *knew* he would receive. To know that you will one day serve as king but have to submit to someone in your position had to be an amazingly humbling experience. Before God gives His children blessings or authority, He tests us over time to determine if we are ready or worthy. David was continually taunted and harassed by Saul, but still kept the faith that what the Lord had appointed him to do would eventually manifest. God was proving and refining his character in the wait. Your Miscarried Joy is a divine circumstance from a God that does not operate according to time.

David, the murderer and adulterer, became a man after God's own heart. Yes, David had some falls during his waiting season and even afterwards, but He allowed God to convert him from the inside out. He had to be pushed, pressed and shaken to successfully reign over the people whom he was called to serve. David reverenced God in everything He did to him and the powerful ways He worked through him. He stood firm on his faith knowing that God was his rock, his fortress, his shield to keep him from harm, a horn of salvation and high above anything he would encounter.

> *"I love you, LORD, my strength. The LORD is my rock, my fortress and my deliverer; my God is my rock, in whom I take refuge, my shield and the horn of my salvation, my stronghold. I called to the LORD, who is worthy of praise, and I have been saved from my enemies." (Psalm 18:1-3 NIV)*

David *became* trusting, devoted, faithful and obedient. *"And it is impossible to please God without faith. Anyone who wants to come to him must believe that God exists and that he rewards those who sincerely seek him" (Hebrews 11:6).* So, for

We must shift

our *focus*

from our current

circumstances

to our future

celebrations,

in faith.

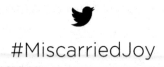

#MiscarriedJoy

David to be called a man after God's own heart, he surely must have been a faithful man even through unbearable circumstances. He pleased God. There are countless others in the bible that exuded great faith resulting in great rewards.

"How much more do I need to say? It would take too long to recount the stories of the faith of Gideon, Barak, Samson, Jephthah, David, Samuel, and all the prophets. By faith these people overthrew kingdoms, ruled with justice, and received what God had promised them. They shut the mouths of lions, quenched the flames of fire, and escaped death by the edge of the sword. Their weakness was turned to strength. They became strong in battle and put whole armies to flight. Women received their loved ones back again from death.

But others were tortured, refusing to turn from God in order to be set free. They placed their hope in a better life after the resurrection. Some were jeered at, and their backs were cut open with whips. Others were chained in prisons. Some died by stoning, some were sawed in half, and others were killed with the sword. Some went about wearing skins of sheep and goats, destitute and oppressed and mistreated. They were too good for this world, wandering over deserts and mountains, hiding in caves and holes in the ground.

All these people earned a good reputation because of their faith, yet none of them received all that God had promised. For God had something better in mind for us, so that they would not reach perfection without us." (Hebrews 11:32-40)

We, too, can experience victory through our faith in Jesus Christ. This is a season of preparation for us. It's a time to truly enjoy and reflect all that God has done. Our faith is not displayed in our ability to wait, but in what we do while we wait.

THE GREAT EXPECTATION

When parents find out they are expecting, they begin to plan. They register for the baby shower gifts, pick out a theme, paint and decorate the room and choose names. They emotionally and excitedly anticipate the arrival of their baby. Women who have not experienced a pregnancy loss may not even consider the worst, but rather focus on the best. In just nine months, they will be holding the greatest blessing of all. Why do they prepare? Because they have faith in God that their baby will be delivered to them. Doubts don't come into play and fear doesn't surface. This is faith! They totally believe and trust that their bodies and the baby in their womb will perform and develop exactly how God planned. The great expectation requires that we stop focusing on the loss and work towards the gains. Not just the blessing of our children, but the blessing of our marriages, our relationships, our careers, our businesses and, most importantly, the callings Jesus Christ has placed on our lives.

For some time after our second miscarriage, I placed a great amount of focus on when, and sometimes if, we would become parents. I dreamed about it and of course it seemed like everyone had a "prophecy" to deliver to me that I would have children. It just became way too much. I vividly remember the day I decided to hand it totally over to God and get on with my life, so to speak. It was a beautiful day, just at the turn from winter to spring. The birds were chirping, the dew was slightly settled on our front grass, the sun was shining, and the perennial flowers in our yard were starting to bud. Then I heard God whisper this to me: "Bloom where you are planted." I had heard this saying before but wondered why God was saying it to me at that moment. It was during a very hard season. I had lost my "good paying, secure, corporate job," we had recently lost our brother, and finding a job was taking way more time than I expected. See, I told you, patience is an area of opportunity for me!

I asked my Father, "Lord, what do you mean by bloom where I am planted?" Then I began to think about the flowers in our yard. They endure so much hard weather throughout the year. When the weather transitions from warm to cool, they begin to die. When the snow arrives, they adapt to the cold, and when spring rolls around, they begin to bud again. Though they are forced to endure hard conditions, they still bloom right where they are planted. They understand that there are seasons in their lifespan, but they adapt and still manage to flourish at the proper time. God wants us to be like these perennial flowers. He wants us to have faith in Him to bring the sun after the rain and the summer after the winter. But even in the storms, He needs us to adapt to the conditions and keep moving forward. This is what I had to do. I had to accept this was a hard season and I could not focus on the pain, but increase my expectation and anticipation of what God was going to do after this. We must shift our focus from our current circumstances to our future celebrations, in faith. God clearly told me to bloom where I am planted in this season, meaning, make the most of it!

We live in Chicago, you can imagine the winters we have in addition to the mighty winds that blow. I love summertime in Chicago! I can't imagine spending the summer months in any other place. I already told you how much I love Lake Michigan! Add to that the beautiful skyline, outdoor festivals, amazing food with rooftop views, boat rides from Navy Pier, and countless other things to do. When I tell you we maximize summers here, that is exactly what I mean. Then there is fall, which is my favorite. But what about the winter? I definitely don't look forward to the cold, dreary and snowy days. But I have learned to enjoy and appreciate every season. Why? Because they are all gifts.

"Every season, God?"
"Yes, My daughter. Every single season."
"Even the hard seasons?"
"Especially the hard seasons."

I've had some very tough seasons in my life, outside of my losses. I'm talking about rock and hard place type of tough! You know, the "God, this can't be my life" type of tough. But do you know what I've learned? It's in these hard places where God works IN you so He can work THROUGH you. These hard places are necessary. They sting, they frustrate you, and may even make you upset with God. Yes, with God! He allows everything that happens in our lives. Every single thing. Since He is such a gracious and loving Father, we know that though it doesn't feel good, it will work out for our good. They say that time flies when you are having fun. So, to make these hard seasons pass faster, let's make the very best of them without whining and complaining. Instead, welcome it full of faith and great joy.

The *hard*

places are

necessary.

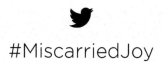

#MiscarriedJoy

My husband and I have learned to enjoy one another and are building a foundation strong enough to endure the extra weight that children will bring. We see the vision of where God is taking us and we are preparing for that. Do we think about our future children? Absolutely we do! In fact, we've stepped out on faith and made purchases for our children. Ask Maurice how many pairs of shoes our son has compared to our daughter? We have also begun financially preparing for children. We believe it will happen, but we can no longer focus on when. If we let our unfulfilled desires consume our thoughts, we will get behind in accomplishing our ultimate purpose. Why? Because whatever you focus on most is what will grow. Whatever you feed, is where you'll feast. Jealously and envy will grow. Impatience will take root. Gratitude will cease and it will become increasingly difficult to focus on the haves, rather than the have nots.

FAITH IN ACTION

There is great power in taking physical actions as a sign of really believing God. Ask the paralytic man who Jesus healed.

"When Jesus returned to Capernaum several days later, the news spread quickly that he was back home. Soon the house where he was staying was so packed with visitors that there was no more room, even outside the door. While he was preaching God's word to them, four men arrived carrying a paralyzed man on a mat. They couldn't bring him to Jesus because of the crowd, so they dug a hole through the roof above his head. Then they lowered the man on his mat, right down in front of Jesus.

Seeing their faith, Jesus said to the paralyzed man, "My child, your sins are forgiven." (Mark 2:1-5)

This man had a need that only Jesus could fulfill. Compassion moved His friends by faith. "If only we can get Him to Jesus!" I imagine this is what they repeatedly yelled as they carried their friend down the streets, around winding roads and through the large crowds. Everything stood in the way of getting him to Jesus. But they went above and beyond to get into the sweet presence of The Healer. It was their faith in action that brought healing to this man. You can go to every infertility specialist, but without faith, their treatments will be unproductive. You need your faith for anything to work! God needs your faith to be activated in this season. What are you doing that shows you really believe God will do this for you?

I have been a Christian for a long time. But let me be honest with you about something. My prayer life sucked! I mean, Whenever I was confronted with a problem, I prayed, but often it was the "God, can you do this?" or "God I need this," prayers. I once felt like I had to pray like the leader of the prayer ministry for my prayers to get to heaven. Oh is that so far from the truth. I knew what faith meant and I believed for everyone else. But when I needed to believe God for me, my faith quickly failed. Why? Because I was a spirit who never had the spiritual experiences necessary to really know, love and trust God.

But my miscarried bundles of joy have absolutely changed my life for the better. I would have never known God as a Comforter until I prayed daily for Him to comfort me. I would have never known the extent of His love until I felt like He didn't love me at all. I would have never known

Him as a healer until I needed an emotional restoration that only He could provide. I would have never been able to truly recognize His voice in this situation of my life until I had no other name to call. But none of this would have been received if I had not believed that God would be all I needed Him to be. So keep spiritually fighting through these hard places, these cold seasons, and the dry, dusty winds that blow. God is there with you and in front of you. You'll come out better than before and you'll learn to appreciate the gift of every season!

Each one of us has been in this season of waiting for various lengths of time. Those who have been waiting for five, ten or even fifteen years may feel like there is no hope. You may be saying, "Well, maybe God doesn't want me to have children." This is a fear statement void of faith. Many of us do this in an attempt to comfort our hurting hearts, but what it really does is send a message to God that we don't believe He is capable of working through the impossible. Since I have been in this season, it seems as if I hear more stories than ever about women who have experienced the loss of a child, or whom are waiting for physical healing in their bodies. One story I heard really touched me. A woman and her husband had been waiting for almost ten years to have children. Do you know what they did? They built a nursery in their home for the arrival of their baby. Yes, the baby who had not been conceived yet. I thought we were doing something buying baby clothes, but this couple should receive the Faith Award!

The woman with the issue of blood was hemorrhaging for twelve years. She had probably visited more physicians than she could count and was left with no additional options. With depleted funds, a lack of energy, hanging on to her last hope, she made her way to Jesus. She had heard He could heal her. She had so much faith that she didn't even need Jesus to touch her. All she needed was to touch the smallest piece of his garment, the hem. Countless people surrounded Jesus. He was on His way to heal Jairus's daughter. It was virtually impossible for her to make her way through the crowds. But her faith gave her the energy to keep moving forward when she needed to lay down. Her faith gave her the motivation to keep going when she wanted to quit. Her faith gave her the strength to fight through the people, to keep her eyes fixed on Jesus and to get close enough to Him to receive her blessing.

"On the other side of the lake the crowds welcomed Jesus, because they had been waiting for him. Then a man named Jairus, a leader of the local synagogue, came and fell at Jesus' feet, pleading with him to come home with him. His only daughter, who was about twelve years old, was dying.

As Jesus went with him, he was surrounded by the crowds. A woman in the crowd had suffered for twelve years with constant bleeding, and she could find no cure. Coming up behind Jesus, she touched the fringe of his robe. Immediately, the bleeding stopped.

"Who touched me?" Jesus asked.

Everyone denied it, and Peter said, "Master, this whole crowd is pressing up against you."

But Jesus said, "Someone deliberately touched me, for I felt healing power go out from me." When the woman realized that she could not stay hidden, she began to tremble and fell to her knees in front of him. The whole crowd heard her explain why she had touched him and that she had been immediately healed. "Daughter," he said to her, "your faith has made you well. Go in peace." (Luke 8:40-48)

She was an ordinary woman who walked in extraordinary faith. After twelve years of suffering, she was ready for a miracle. So she consecrated herself, elevated her prayer life, filled her heart with The Word of God and walked towards Jesus. She wasn't concerned with the blood trail that followed her as she made her way to Him. She didn't care about the gossipers nor the people who thought she was crazy. She needed God to turn her situation totally around. People were pushing and pressing into Him, but He stopped just for her. She needed Him to show Himself faithful in her life. Jesus did what no doctor could do. You, my sister, have an issue. I have an issue. We need God to turn this around for us because we believe that our desire to become mothers was placed in our hearts with the beautiful hands of God. He is just waiting on our faith!

"The fundamental fact of existence is that this trust in God, this faith, is the firm foundation under everything that makes life worth living. It's our handle on what we can't see. The act of faith is what distinguished our ancestors, set them above the crowd. By faith, we see the world called into existence by God's Word, what we see created by what we don't see." (Hebrews 11:1-3 MSG)

There you have it! Faith, not fear, not worry, not doubt, but faith is what makes life worth living. Your life is abundantly blessed because you have the breath of life in you. Your life is blessed because most of what you have asked God for has been rewarded to you. Your life is blessed because He has closed doors to protect you. Your life is blessed because by faith, everything you desire will be delivered to you. But you have to keep living a life of great expectation. Your babies will be conceived soon, so confess with faith, "We are Expecting!"

CHAPTER 10

The Birthing Room

I s there a lot going on in your life on top of this tough season being in the back of your mind? Has this season seemed like one where you could possibly be in the midst of a famine? Do you feel like everything you need to get to the next place is being stripped away from you? Are you familiar with the saying, "If it isn't one thing, it's another!" I know that a baby isn't the only thing you are believing God for and it just may not be the only thing you've recently miscarried or are having challenges conceiving. Has a loss or delay in other areas of your life added to those feelings of frustration? Do you have moments when you feel broken? Crushed? Shattered? Confused? Hurt? Abandoned? Distraught? Guess who else can understand the place we are in? Naomi. We often focus on the story of Ruth and the journey to her Boaz, but there is a powerful revelation that we can obtain as we look deeper into the life of Naomi.

Naomi, whose name means "my joy, bliss or the pleasantness of Jehovah," was a woman who experienced the

God uses the *tragic*

pieces of our lives to

build, restore and to

resurrect those places

we *thought*

were once dead.

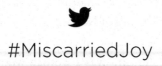

#MiscarriedJoy

very opposite of her name. She was married to Elimelech, who belonged to one of the most well-off families in Israel. Let's just say she "married up" as it relates to finances. She was sitting pretty comfortable with her new husband with no care or concern within her distance. And then circumstances took a turn for the worse. Israel suffered a severe famine as a consequence to the sin that was so prevalent throughout their land. Elimelech did what any good, protective man would probably do in a similar situation. He packed his family up and moved to a land where resources were bountiful. That land was Moab. They went from being citizens to foreigners. While moving would have seemed like the right thing to do, it was never mentioned that they prayed and asked God for guidance. Don't we forget to do that sometimes, too? Or maybe it's just me. I guess Elimelech forgot God's promise that even in the days of famine, His people would be satisfied.

"Even strong young lions sometimes go hungry, but those who trust in the LORD will lack no good thing." (Psalm 34:10)

This is a powerful lesson, because even in the midst of what seems like a deep loss or famine in your season, God is more than able to provide all *you* need to not just survive, but to truly thrive. He has more than enough peace, patience, joy, and strength to pull you out of where you are today. The famine may not immediately go away, but it won't feel like a famine to you! So in a haste to move, they ended up encountering a land full of heathens after leaving a land full of God's people. Be careful of what moves you make out of emotion. You could end up in a worse situation than you were in before.

Poor Naomi. Through her submission to her husband, she ended up in a land where she didn't know anyone. It was just her, Elimelech and their two sons – Mahlon and Kilion. Being in search of a better life left her with a bitter life. Shortly after moving, she lost her husband. She was now a single mom, raising two sons in a land full of people who had opposite beliefs of her. What a difficult time this must have been for her. She didn't ask for any of this, but she had to learn how to endure. She had no other choice but to pull her strength from the Almighty Father. She raised them into what I assume were respectable young men. Instead of her sons growing up and working to provide for their mom, they married Moabite women. The Jewish law strictly forbade marriage outside of their native land. It seems like she ended up leaving a bad situation for a worse one.

I imagine Naomi felt like us and any others who have miscarried their purpose or destiny. She felt alone among a land of many. She may have felt alone even in the company of her sons, but still showed great strength. She possibly felt abandoned by God. How could He not come and sweep her out of this grief-stricken situation, especially since she never stopped serving Him wholeheartedly. How could God forget about this loyal daughter, Naomi? Things got worse before they got better. Her sons died and she was left with two widowed daughters-in-law, Ruth and Orpah. What in the world was she was supposed to do now? She was in the middle of nowhere, around pagans and idol worshippers. She was left with...nothing! And who did she blame? God! That's right. She felt as if He was responsible for the agony she was experiencing.

"The Lord Himself has raised His fist against me."
(Ruth 1:13b)

Naomi had finally realized the mistake they made by fleeing their home land. Once Naomi had received word that the Lord brought prosperity upon the land of Judah, she decided to return home and take her daughters with her. But as they began to travel, Naomi realized she had nothing left to pour into them, no wealth to give them and definitely no sons left for them to marry.

> *"Then Naomi heard in Moab that the LORD had blessed his people in Judah by giving them good crops again. So Naomi and her daughters-in-law got ready to leave Moab to return to her homeland. With her two daughters-in-law she set out from the place where she had been living, and they took the road that would lead them back to Judah." (Ruth 1:6-7)*

She was left with one choice; thus, commissioned them to return home. Orpah agreed and went back to her home while Ruth refused to leave Naomi's side. So they returned to Bethlehem together. When Naomi left Judah, she was rich, but returned poor. She was full of life and love but returned feeling abandoned and bitter. Because of this, her eyes were blind to the plan God was unfolding right before her. Our brokenness has a tendency to prevent us from seeing what God is building in our lives. That is why we must constantly renew our minds and walk in faith even when frustration gets the very best of who we are.

> *"Don't call me Naomi," she responded. "Instead, call me Mara for the Almighty has made life very bitter for me.*

If you *allow* God to

privately *develop*

you, He will publicly

bless you.

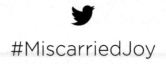

I went away full, but the LORD has brought me home empty. Why call me Naomi when the LORD has caused me to suffer and the Almighty has sent such tragedy upon me?"
(Ruth 1:20-21)

It was through Naomi that Ruth met Boaz. Their marriage and the birth of their children restored Naomi's lineage, which she thought had died forever back in Moab. God uses the tragic pieces of our lives to build, restore and to resurrect those places we thought were once dead. The feelings of loss turn into moments of joy. Sometimes, when we are in our darkest hours, all we can see is bleakness, hopelessness and sorrow. We fail to see God at work and His light shining into the miscarried situations of our lives. God did not abandon Naomi or allow her to be destroyed. He extends that same grace to us as well. His plan to restore her hope and rebuild her future started in the very person she wanted to let go – Ruth. The plan was fully manifested when Boaz found his good thing. In the times when Naomi felt alone, God was carrying her through.

BEAUTY FOR ASHES

"The Spirit of the Sovereign LORD is upon me, for the LORD has anointed me to bring good news to the poor. He has sent me to comfort the brokenhearted and to proclaim that captives will be released and prisoners will be freed. He has sent me to tell those who mourn that the time of the LORD's favor has come, and with it, the day of God's anger against their enemies. To all who mourn in Israel, he will give a crown of beauty for ashes, a joyous blessing instead of mourning, festive praise instead of

despair. In their righteousness, they will be like great oaks that
the LORD has planted for his own glory." (Isaiah 61:1-3)

I know how you may feel in those moments you are alone.
I have been there and still visit those places from time to
time. And it is not always by accident either. Yes, sometimes I
journey there all on my own. I allow my emotions to get the
best of me and take me to that broken place. The place where
I am constantly reminded of my loss and disappointments.
The missing pieces to this Fitzgerald Family puzzle often
take me there again and again. Your emotions have probably
taken you to the same place.

> When you receive the news of another friend expecting.
> When you get less than favorable news from your doctor.
> When the pregnancy test is negative once again.
> When you don't get the job you've prayed for.
> When those closest to you let you down.
> When you don't know which way to turn.
> When you're constantly reminded that you are still waiting.
> It's taxing. Overwhelming. Not a thrill ride in any way.

But Jesus can empathize with us. He knew what it felt like
to be crushed. He feels your pain because He Himself carried
it. All the way to the cross. He didn't want to, but because it
was the perfect will of His Father, he completed the mission
against his own will.

> *"He told them, "My soul is crushed with grief to the point*
> *of death. Stay here and keep watch with me." He went*
> *on a little farther and fell to the ground. He prayed, that*
> *if it were possible, the awful hour awaiting him might*

pass him by. "Abba, Father," he cried out, "everything is possible for you. Please take this cup of suffering away from me. Yet I want your will to be done, not mine."
(Mark 14:34-36)

Jesus wrestled with His divine appointment with pain too. He felt what we feel and He wanted God to take away the pain. But for our Savior, it got worse before it got better. He was beat, bruised, and killed for the chastisement of our sin. But God's purpose was to use His son all for His glory. It was a necessary crushing. There wasn't anything He could do to avoid it. Because of His sacrifice, you, me and so many others have received the free, beautiful and priceless gift of salvation. What He gave birth to was so much more than the pain He had to endure.

I remember watching the show *Amazing Race*. There was an obstacle where each team was given a humongous tub of grapes. One of the team members had to remove their shoes, get inside of it and stomp on the grapes as hard as they possibly could. With each large stomp came the tiniest bit of juice. But the more she stomped, the more juice was extracted. Envision being those grapes. Imagine being stomped on, bruised for reasons you don't understand, crushed, and broken. Oh wait, that is where we have been, isn't it? And it may even be where you stand now. It doesn't feel good, but those grapes have the tendency to produce the sweetest wine. In order for them to be useful and fulfill their purpose, they had to go through the agitation.

With tears in my eyes, I connect with you one more time. This season can make you or it can break you. But you can also choose to be the clay molded by the Master Potter. Firing is the process of bringing clay up to a high temperature so that it can be molded into whatever the potter chooses. You, my sister, are in the firing process. Firing clay transforms it from its very soft beginning into a new ceramic substance that is strong, tough and able to be preserved for a very long time. God's spiritual process of preserving us will feel as if we are being pressed from every side.

> *"We are pressed on every side by troubles, but we are not crushed. We are perplexed, but not driven to despair. We are hunted down, but never abandoned by God. we get knocked down, but are not destroyed. Through suffering, our bodies continue to share in the death of Jesus so that the life of Jesus may also be seen in our bodies." (2 Corinthians 4:8-10)*

Pregnancy isn't always easy. There is some discomfort and lots of pushing involved. But I prophesy to you now that you are about to give birth to something. God has something He needs to conceive in you and it's much bigger than the baby you've been praying for. It's bigger than the losses you've suffered. It's bigger than anything you can imagine. So, while you're in the birthing room, take the stones being thrown at you and build something. Build a life of gratitude, a house of grace, a foundation of trust, and a path of love. Yes, use the really hard places and build. That's faith in action. That's making lemons out of lemonade. That's taking everything the enemy meant for evil and turning it around for your good. We cannot let Satan win this war. We had the victory before it started and we must hold on to it. Our attitude determines our outcome.

"It's time to push!"

Appreciate the

beauty in the ashes,

the *blessing*

in the discomfort,

and the *wonder*

in the waiting.

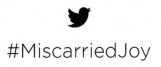

#MiscarriedJoy

Whew! A great sigh of relief is emitted from the mother who has been laboring and in pain for hours, maybe even days. The moment she has been greatly awaiting is almost here. All she has to do is push. The worst is over and the greatest moment ever is about to take place. Out of nowhere comes a strength she's never known. A few hours or even minutes before, she questioned if she could take any more pain. She didn't want to feel another contraction, she was tired of hearing her husband say, "You are doing well, honey. Keep up the good work," while he stands there fully clothed, not having to bear every part of his body to strangers and full of scrumptious food rather than ice chips! Her whole attitude changes once she realizes the last part of this journey is about to end.

So, she grabs the rails on the bed, pulls herself up and pushes with every muscle in her body. After just five to ten pushes, she hears the most joyous sound she could ever imagine – the crying of *her* baby. The instant skin to skin contact happens and every pain she felt over the past several hours has been erased from her mind. It was all worth it and she would do it again just to give birth to the blessing she had been praying for even prior to the positive pregnancy test.

But before the joy, there were those very ugly moments. I know the occurrences in this season aren't the ones we openly share or tweet about. These are the very private pieces of your life. And if you allow God to privately develop you, He will publicly bless you. No one wants to experience a broken-heart, but the birthing place is where God pieces it all back together. The other side of this is oh so sweet. It's the manifestation of His promises to you. Your purpose has crowned and you are finally about to give birth to the vision you've been praying for. You may feel as if you've been to the bottom of hell and back. Maybe more than once. But the baby (whatever or whomever this baby may be in your life) you will soon hold in your hands will be immeasurably worth the pain you'll soon forget. But I caution you. Don't forget God on the other side.

The God who brought you through.
The God who dried your tears.
The God who heard your heart.
The God who calmed your fears.
The God who held you tight in the lonely, dark nights.
The God who relieved your pain.
The God who allowed you to be broken, but not destroyed.

Yes, Him! He is altogether lovely, altogether worthy and altogether wonderful. He is sovereign. He reigns above anything in our lives. He is trustworthy. He is dependable. He is good. No, He is amazing! These times will become a mere memory, but be sure to use this season for His glory. Don't be the married woman who forgets what it was like to be single. Don't be the corporate woman who forgets what it was like to be without opportunity. Don't be the friend who forgets what it was like to be lonely. Don't forget what you've been through just because it's over. Use it.

To glorify God.
To help others.
To strengthen your sister.
To keep your brother.
To share how loving, thoughtful and kind the God we serve is to His people.

Our *brokenness*

has a tendency to

prevent us from

seeing what God is

building in

our lives.

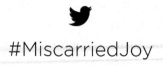

#MiscarriedJoy

You have carried this assignment to full term and now, it is time to...

Push! Push! Push! Push!

Keep pushing through the pain. This will not be a premature birth. Your due time has come. Give birth with great contentment. You are out of the waiting room and your delay has been perfectly divine. It's labor and delivery time in the birthing room. Keep pushing, my sister. Great destiny is birthed out of great pain! The greater the test, the greater the blessing. You have to push to give birth to the baby you desperately want to meet! Appreciate the beauty in the ashes, the blessing in the discomfort, and the wonder in the waiting. Please remember that it is not about the destination but the journey along the way.

Congratulations! In faith, your promise has been manifested.

A Note from Tanika

Sister,

Thank you so much for allowing me to share the transparency of my journey with you. Writing this book was so difficult for me. I am a very private person, so when God told me to share my story with the whole world, I was a bit hesitant, yet obedient. I have always felt like the testimonies in my life weren't big enough to have an impact on the lives of others. I now know there is always another person that we have the ability to help. I never imagined God would choose me to endure such pain and then use that pain for the purpose of helping women all over the world. It is my prayer that when you close this book, you close it with bouts of encouragement, joy, laughter and a faith that is stronger than it was when you read the first word on the very first page.

Though we may not have met in person, I want you to know that God has given me an unexplainable compassion for what you are going through. I am you. I know your hurts, your frustration and the emotional roller coaster you involuntarily ride. I pray you feel my love on every page of every chapter. I needed this book. I needed to release all the pinned up grief that I never knew was there. I needed to talk to women like you who understand my tears. I needed to be reminded that God has a purpose and a plan even when I don't understand. I needed to take my prayer life to a different level and, most of all, this wilderness experience has led me to fully walk in my purpose. So, my dear sister, I want to thank you for your time, attention, your conversations, your laughs and your tears.

I want to leave you with a few special tools that have helped Maurice and me to keep smiling during our walk through this dry, dusty desert land. We confess what we believe God will do for us. I am fully convinced that what we release into the atmosphere will manifest in the earth. And since you, too, are awaiting your precious bundles of joy, I want to share our confession of faith. Maurice and I confess this together daily. Please use this confession and feel free to make it your own. I want you to email me or send me a message on Facebook when your bundle of joy arrives. I am joining my faith with yours and I want to know about the manifestation of God's amazing promises in your life.

With Love,
Tanika Fitzgerald

A Faith Confession for Our Bundles of Joy

Lord, we thank you for this child You are forming in my womb. According to Jeremiah 1:5, we thank You that You already know him/her before they are conceived. We confess that this child will be set apart for a mighty purpose in Your Kingdom. As a disciple of Jesus Christ, we have the keys of the kingdom of heaven and whatever we bind on earth will be bound in heaven. In the same way, whatever we loose on earth, shall be loosed in heaven. God, we bind the spirit of fear about our future pregnancies due to the losses we have experienced. We bind all negative thoughts and emotions.

I will not miscarry nor be barren, and we will give birth to healthy babies (Exodus 23:25-26). I will not be anxious about my pregnancy or delivery, and peace in my heart and mind shall be my portion. Because we worship you in every area of our lives, Your abundant blessings are upon my food and water, and everything I eat or drink. You have taken all morning, afternoon and evening sickness from me. I will not have nausea, food aversions, lack of energy or any other conditions that will keep me from walking in the Kingdom assignments you have given me during my pregnancy. Thank you for bestowing upon me all deep blessing of the breasts and of the womb (Genesis 49:25).

Satan is defeated and he will never be able to touch our babies (Isaiah 44:24). All of our children shall be taught about the Lord and great shall be their peace and undisturbed composure (Isaiah 54:13).

Lord, You have upheld me from the time of my birth. You brought me from my mother's womb at Your perfectly appointed time. Father, I thank You that You will also bring forth my babies at your perfect hour and I will praise you continually. (Psalm 71:6)

I have faith that my labor will be supernatural, pain free and without any need for medication. There will be no complications and our babies will come into this world without sickness, deformities, disorders and the like. I shall not labor in vain or have trouble delivering my children, for I and my offspring are the seed of the blessed from the Lord. (Isaiah 65:23)

I thank you that even my breasts will produce an overflow of milk to nurse my babies from the day they are born.

We will commit our children back to You and raise them according to Your Word. They will pray, know Jesus and love You with all of their heart. May you protect them from all harm and may they serve You all the days of their lives.

I praise You that the creation of my babies is wonderful. All the days of their lives are written in Your book before they take place or even before their substance has been formed (Psalm 139:13-16).

We claim all of this by faith in Jesus' name. Amen!

Scriptures of Comfort in Infertility & Pregnancy Loss

Exodus 23:26 (NLT) *There will be no miscarriages or infertility in your land, and I will give you long, full lives.*	***1 Samuel 1:27-28 (NIV)*** *"I prayed for this child, and the LORD has granted me what I asked of him. So now I give him to the LORD. For his whole life he will be given over to the LORD." And he worshiped the LORD there."*
Psalm 23:4 *"Even though I walk through the valley of the shadow of death, I fear no evil; for Thou art with me."*	***Psalm 34:18*** *"The LORD is close to the brokenhearted and saves those who are crushed in spirit."*
Ecclesiastes 11:5 *"As you do not know the path of the wind, or how the body is formed in a mother's womb so you cannot understand the work of God, the Maker of all things."*	***Psalm 119:50*** *"My comfort in my suffering is this: Your promise preserves my life."*

Psalm 126:6 *"Those who go out weeping, carrying seed to sow, will return with songs of joy, carrying sheaves with them."*	**Isaiah 49:15** *"Can a mother forget the baby at her breast and have no compassion on the child she has borne? Though she may forget, I will not forget you!"*
James 1:17 *"Every good and perfect gift is from above, coming down from the Father of the heavenly lights, who does not change like shifting shadows."*	**Psalms 73:26** *"My flesh and my heart may fail, but God is the strength of my heart and my portion forever."*
Isaiah 41:10 *"Fear not, for I am with you; be not dismayed, for I am your God; I will strengthen you, I will help you, I will uphold you with my righteous right hand."*	**Matthew 11:28-30** *"Come to me, all who labor and are heavy laden, and I will give you rest. Take my yoke upon you, and learn from me, for I am gentle and lowly in heart, and you will find rest for your souls. For my yoke is easy, and my burden is light."*

John 14:27	*2 Corinthians 12:9*
"Peace I leave with you; my peace I give to you. Not as the world gives do I give to you. Let not your hearts be troubled, neither let them be afraid."	"But he said to me, "My grace is sufficient for you, for my power is made perfect in weakness." Therefore I will boast all the more gladly of my weaknesses, so that the power of Christ may rest upon me."
Matthew 5:4	*Romans 8:18-19*
"Blessed are those who mourn for they shall be comforted."	"I consider that our present sufferings are not worth comparing with the glory that will be revealed in us. For the creation waits in eager expectation for the children of God to be revealed."

Romans 8:28	2 Corinthians 1:3-7
"We know that in everything God works for good with those who love him, who are called according to His purpose."	*"Praise be to the God and Father of our Lord Jesus Christ, the Father of compassion and the God of all comfort, who comforts us in all our troubles, so that we can comfort those in any trouble with the comfort we ourselves receive from God. For just as we share abundantly in the sufferings of Christ, so also our comfort abounds through Christ. If we are distressed, it is for your comfort and salvation; if we are comforted, it is for your comfort, which produces in you patient endurance of the same sufferings we suffer. And our hope for you is firm, because we know that just as you share in our sufferings, so also you share in our comfort."*

Notes

1. "Miscarriage: Signs, Symptoms, Treatment and Prevention." *American Pregnancy Association*, Accessed March 7, 2016, *http://americanpregnancy.org/pregnancy-complications/miscarriage.*
2. "Miscarriage: Signs, Symptoms, Treatment and Prevention." *American Pregnancy Association*, Accessed March 7, 2016, *http://americanpregnancy.org/pregnancy-complications/miscarriage.*
3. "National Survey of Family Growth, Centers for Disease Control and Prevention [CDC] 2006-2010", Accessed March 7, 2016, *http://www.cdc.gov/nchs/nvss/births.htm.*
4. "Vine's Greek New Testament Dictionary", Accessed March 15, 2016, *http://gospelhall.org/bible/bible.php?search=PROMISE&dict=vine&lang=english*
5. "Experience His Power – Power to Change", Accessed March 16, 2016, *https://powertochange.com/experience/sex-love/prayinghusband/*
6. "Experience His Power – Power to Change", Accessed March 16, 2016, *https://powertochange.com/experience/sex-love/prayinghusband/*
7. "Merriam Webster Online Dictionary." Accessed March 16, 2016, *http://www.merriam-webster.com/dictionary/peace*

8. "Pearls.com – How Pearls are formed." Accessed March 21, 2016, *http://www.pearls.com/pages/how-pearls-are-formed*

9. "Behind the Name – Zechariah." Accessed, March 21, 2016, *http://www.behindthename.com/name/zechariah*

10. "Behind the Name – Zechariah." Accessed, March 21, 2016, *http://www.behindthename.com/name/elizabeth*

11. "AZ Quotes, Author's Quotes," Accessed March 29, 2016, *http://www.azquotes.com/quote/864603*

About the Author

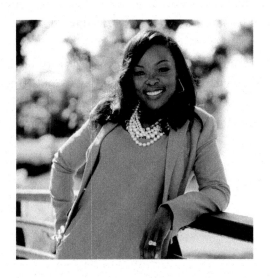

Tanika Fitzgerald is a lover of Christ, a wife to her husband Maurice, a loving daughter and sister. She is passionate about equipping women to grow spiritually, live balanced lives and helping them to be ARMED for victory in every area of life. Tanika has been called to minister to others through her passion and gift of writing to inspire women all over the globe. She is also the visionary behind ARMED Magazine – a publication created to "Spiritually Equip you for Victory in Battle." Her inspirational writing has been featured in numerous publications including *Hope for Women Magazine, Black and Married with Kids* and more. Tanika has also interviewed powerful voices in the Christian Community including, Lady Serita Jakes, Sheryl Brady, Charles Jenkins, Earnest Pugh and more!

Tanika is a woman who is passionate about her relationship with Jesus Christ, family, giving to others, laughter, having fun and enjoying every moment that life brings!

Website: If you enjoyed *Miscarried Joy,* get equipped with additional resources at *www.miscarriedjoy.com*

To Learn more about Tanika, connect with her daily and follow the details of her journey to motherhood:
Blog: *www.tanikafitzgerald.com*
Facebook: *www.facebook.com/tanikafitzgerald*
Instagram: @tanikafitzgerald
Twitter: @TR_Fitzgerald

CPSIA information can be obtained
at www.ICGtesting.com
Printed in the USA
LVOW01s1451240217
525373LV00009B/1052/P